LEARNING CENTRE LIBRARY
ROYAL BLACKBURN HOSPITAL

10588

Books are to be returned on or before
the last date below.

D1389405

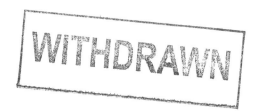
WITHDRAWN

BLACKBURN LEARNING CENTRE
LIBRARY

B14107

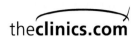

OTOLARYNGOLOGIC CLINICS
OF NORTH AMERICA

Oral Cancer

GUEST EDITOR
Arlen D. Meyers, MD, MBA

April 2006 • Volume 39 • Number 2

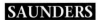

An Imprint of Elsevier, Inc.
PHILADELPHIA   LONDON   TORONTO   MONTREAL   SYDNEY   TOKYO

W.B. SAUNDERS COMPANY
A Division of Elsevier Inc.

1600 John F. Kennedy Boulevard, Suite 1800, Philadelphia, PA 19103–2899

http://www.theclinics.com

THE OTOLARYNGOLOGIC CLINICS	Volume 39, Number 2
OF NORTH AMERICA	ISSN 0030–6665
April 2006	ISBN 1-4160-3586-9
Editor: Joanne Husovski	

Copyright © 2006 Elsevier Inc. All rights reserved. No part of this publication may be reproduced or transmitted in any form or by any means, electronic or mechanical, including photocopy, recording, or any information retrieval system, without written permission from the Publisher.

Single photocopies of single articles may be made for personal use as allowed by national copyright laws. Permission of the Publisher and payment of a fee is required for all other photocopying, including multiple or systematic copying, copying for advertising or promotional purposes, resale, and all forms of document delivery. Special rates are available for educational institutions that wish to make photocopies for non-profit educational classroom use. Permissions may be sought directly from Elsevier's Rights Department in Philadelphia, PA, USA; phone: (+1) 215 239 3804, fax: (+1) 215 239 3805, e-mail: healthpermissions@elsevier.com. Requests may also be completed online via the Elsevier homepage (http://www.elsevier.com/locate/permissions). In the USA, users may clear permissions and make payments through the Copyright Clearance Center, Inc., 222 Rosewood Drive, Danvers, MA 01923, USA; phone: (978) 750-8400, fax: (978) 750-4744, and in the UK through the Copyright Licensing Agency Rapid Clearance Service (CLARCS), 90 Tottenham Court Road, London W1P 0LP, UK; phone: (+44) 171 436 5931; fax: (+44) 171 436 3986. Other countries may have a local reprographic rights agency for payments.

Reprints. For copies of 100 or more, of articles in this publication, please contact the Commercial Reprints Department, Elsevier Inc., 360 Park Avenue South, New York, New York 10010-1710. Tel. (212) 633-3813; Fax: (212) 462-1935; email: reprints@elsevier.com

The ideas and opinions expressed in *The Otolaryngologic Clinics of North America* do not necessarily reflect those of the Publisher. The Publisher does not assume any responsibility for any injury and/or damage to persons or property arising out of or related to any use of the material contained in this periodical. The reader is advised to check the appropriate medical literature and the product information currently provided by the manufacturer of each drug to be administered to verify the dosage, the method and duration of administration, or contraindications. It is the responsibility of the treating physician or other health care professional, relying on independent experience and knowledge of the patient, to determine drug dosages and the best treatment for the patient. Mention of any product in this issue should not be construed as endorsement by the contributors, editors, or the Publisher of the product or manufacturers' claims.

The Otolaryngologic Clinics of North America (ISSN 0030–6665) is published bimonthly by W.B. Saunders, 360 Park Avenue South, New York, NY 10010-1710. Months of publication are February, April, June, August, October, and December. Business and Editorial Offices: 1600 John F. Kennedy Blvd., Suite 1800, Philadelphia, PA 19103-2899. Accounting and Circulation Offices: 6277 Sea Harbor Drive, Orlando, FL 32887-4800. Periodicals postage paid at New York, NY and additional mailing offices. Subscription price is $205.00 per year (US individuals), $370.00 per year (US institutions), $100.00 per year (US student/resident), $270.00 per year (Canadian individuals), $455.00 per year (Canadian institutions), $285.00 per year (international individuals), $455.00 per year (international institutions), $145.00 per year (international & Canadian student/resident). Foreign air speed delivery is included in all *Clinics*' subscription prices. All prices are subject to change without notice. **POSTMASTER:** Send address changes to *The Otolaryngologic Clinics of North America*, Elsevier Periodicals Customer Service, 6277 Sea Harbor Drive, Orlando, FL 32887-4800. **Customer Service: 1-800-654-2452 (US). From outside the US, call 407-345-4000.**

The Otolaryngologic Clinics of North America is also published in Spanish by McGraw-Hill Interamericana Editores S.A., P.O. Box 5-237, 06500 Mexico D.F., Mexico.

The Otolaryngologic Clinics of North America is covered in *Index Medicus, Current Contents/Clinical Medicine, Excerpta Medica, BIOSIS, Science Citation Index,* and *ISI/BIOMED.*

Printed in the United States of America.

GUEST EDITOR

ARLEN D. MEYERS, MD, MBA, Professor, Department of Otolaryngology, University of Colorado Health Sciences Center, Denver, Colorado

CONTRIBUTORS

ARI BALLONOFF, MD, Resident, Department of Radiation Oncology, University of Colorado Health Sciences Center, Aurora, Colorado

KEVIN S. BROWN, MD, Assistant Professor of Medicine, Division of Hematology and Oncology, University of Colorado Health Sciences Center and Denver Health Medical Center, Denver, Colorado

JOHN P. CAMPANA, MD, Assistant Professor, Department of Otolaryngology, University of Colorado Health Sciences Center, Denver, Colorado

CHANGHU CHEN, MD, Assistant Professor, Department of Radiation Oncology, University of Colorado Health Sciences Center, Aurora, Colorado

ROBERT O. GREER, DDS, ScD, Professor and Chair, Division of Oral and Maxillofacial Pathology, University of Colorado School of Dentistry, University of Colorado Health Sciences Center; Professor of Pathology and Medicine, University of Colorado School of Medicine, University of Colorado Health Sciences Center, Denver, Colorado

MADELEINE A. KANE, MD, PhD, Professor of Medicine, Division of Medical Oncology, University of Colorado Health Sciences Center and Denver Veterans Affairs Medical Center, Denver, Colorado

MICHAEL E. KUPFERMAN, MD, Fellow, Department of Head and Neck Surgery, M. D. Anderson Cancer Center of the University of Texas, Houston, Texas

JOHN D. MCDOWELL, DDS, MS, Associate Professor, Department of Diagnostic and Biological Sciences; Chair, Division of Oral Diagnosis; and Director, Oral Medicine and Forensic Sciences, University of Colorado School of Dentistry; Dental Consultant, Mountain-Plains AIDS Education and Training Center, University of Colorado School of Medicine, Denver, Colorado

ARLEN D. MEYERS, MD, MBA, Professor, Department of Otolaryngology, University of Colorado Health Sciences Center, Denver, Colorado

ALAN R. MICKELSON, PhD, Associate Professor, Department of Electrical and Computer Engineering, University of Colorado at Boulder, Boulder, Colorado

ERIC H. MILLER, DDS, Associate Professor, School of Dentistry, University of Colorado Health Sciences Center; Director, General Practice Residency, University Hospital, Denver, Colorado

JEFFREY N. MYERS, MD, PhD, Associate Professor and Deputy Chair for Academic Programs, Department of Head and Neck Surgery, M. D. Anderson Cancer Center of the University of Texas, Houston, Texas

JONATHAN M. OWENS, MD, Department of Otolaryngology-Head and Neck Surgery, University of Colorado Health Sciences Center, Denver, Colorado

WOUNJHANG PARK, PhD, Assistant Professor, Department of Electrical & Computer Engineering, University of Colorado, Boulder, Colorado; University of Colorado Cancer Center, Aurora, Colorado

AUBREY I. QUINN, BS, Educational Consultant, School of Dentistry, University of Colorado Health Sciences Center, Denver, Colorado

DAVID RABEN, MD, Associate Professor, Department of Radiation Oncology, University of Colorado Health Sciences Center, Aurora, Colorado

PRAIRIE NEELEY ROBINSON, MD, Resident Physician, Department of Otolaryngology, University of Colorado Health Sciences Center, Denver, Colorado

DAVID RUBINSTEIN, MD, Department of Radiology, University of Colorado Health Sciences Center, Denver, Colorado

LAURA LEE SIMON, MD, Castle Rock, Colorado

Learning Centre
Library

Barcode: TB14107

Class No: 616.99431 ORA

STAMPS ✓

TRIGGER ✓

CLASS ✓

SPINE ✓

LEARNING CENTRE LIBRARY
ROYAL BLACKBURN HOSPITAL

ORAL CANCER

CONTENTS

> Significant advances have been made in understanding the mech-
> anisms that contribute to carcinogenesis in oral cavity squamous
> cell carcinoma (OCSCC). This progress has led to the development
> of therapeutic strategies that target dysregulated processes in the
> tumor microenvironment. It is important for those caring for pa-
> tients who have OCSCC to have a firm background in tumor biol-
> ogy, because many future therapies will be based on this complex
> panorama of cellular physiology. This article focuses on the current
> knowledge of the molecular processes that underlie tumorigenesis
> and metastasis in OCSCC.

> Oral mucous membranes and the surrounding structures are largely
> composed of stratified squamous epithelium that is supported
> by a fibrous connective tissue lamina propria and a submucosa of
> fibroadipose tissue. Minor salivary glands, nerves, and capillaries
> course abundantly throughout the supporting collagen and fibro-
> fatty submucosa. Premalignant and malignant lesions arise most
> frequently from epithelium, and these epithelial lesions ultimately
> account for 95% of all cancers of the oral cavity. Malignant neopla-
> sia of bone, cartilage, salivary glands, and connective tissue and
> those of lymphoproliferative derivatives are far less common oc-
> currences in the oral cavity. Malignant neoplasms can and do arise
> from the tooth germ apparatus, but neoplasms of odontogenic ele-
> ments are rare and are not included in this discussion.

An Overview of Epidemiology and Common Risk Factors for Oral Squamous Cell Carcinoma

John D. McDowell

Understanding the epidemiologic picture and the risk factors for oral cancer can help identify and treat patients at risk for oral cancers. Early diagnosis of an oral cancer continues to be critically important to achieving a favorable prognosis. Absent a diagnosis of oral/pharyngeal cancer, an effective treatment plan is impossible. Discovering a potentially malignant or malignant lesion and through biopsy reaching a diagnosis for the lesion begins by performing an examination with the purpose of detecting oral/pharyngeal lesions. Physicians, dentists and other health care providers should be performing the oral cancer screening examination on a routine basis for all of their patients.

Early Diagnosis of Oral Cavity Cancers

Prairie Neeley Robinson and Alan R. Mickelson

Dentists, primary care physicians, and otolaryngologists should continue to perform complete oral cavity examinations and should be aware of high-risk populations for oral cavity carcinomas. Oral cavity carcinoma is the sixth most common cancer and is often detected in later stages. By using the modalities of physical examination, brush biopsies, vital staining, and spectral analysis, it is hoped that more cancers will be detected at an early stage, decreasing the morbidity and mortality of oral cavity tumors.

Imaging of Oral Cancer

Laura Lee Simon and David Rubinstein

This article reviews imaging modalities commonly used to evaluate oral cavity cancers and their metastases to lymph nodes. It discusses how the studies are performed and their relative merits. It also presents new techniques for evaluating these neoplasms.

Dental Considerations in the Management of Head and Neck Cancer Patients

Eric H. Miller and Aubrey I. Quinn

This article emphasizes the need for a timely dental consult early in the process of the head and neck cancer patient's treatment. Nonrestorable diseased teeth should be removed before radiation and chemotherapy. The primary survey of the patient should include an examination of the oral cavity, noting the state of the dentition and periodontal tissues. Complications commonly seen in patient's undergoing radiotherapy may be reduced, improving the patient's quality of life. Optimizing the patient's oral health benefits the patient's postsurgical and postirradiation course. The dental health care professional can serve an important role in the overall outcome of the patient's care.

FORTHCOMING ISSUES

RECENT ISSUES

The Clinics are now available online!

Access your subscription at
www.theclinics.com

ELSEVIER
SAUNDERS

Otolaryngol Clin N Am
39 (2006) xi–xii

OTOLARYNGOLOGIC
CLINICS
OF NORTH AMERICA

Preface

Oral Cancer

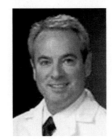

Arlen D. Meyers, MD, MBA
Guest Editor

Oral cancer is the sixth most common cancer in the United States. Each year, 30,000 Americans and more than 300,000 people worldwide will be diagnosed as having oral cancer, and 8000 to 10,000 deaths in the United States will result. Unfortunately, although significant advances have been made in the diagnosis and treatment of oral cancer, the survival rate has not meaningfully changed in 30 years.

This issue reviews recent advances in the approach to oral cancer. An experienced interdisciplinary team from MD Anderson Cancer Hospital and the University of Colorado Cancer Center describes how new technologies in dentistry, cell biology, engineering, imaging, and computer science are finding their way into the mainstream of oral cancer management.

Despite our better understanding of the cell biology and behavior of oral cancer, significant challenges lie ahead if we are to improve survival and reduce the morbidity from treatment. Present techniques for the early detection of early cancer are not sufficiently sensitive or specific. One half of patients still present with advanced-stage disease. Despite the description of hundreds of biomarkers, none are universally accepted in biostaging. A disturbing number of patients are developing oral cancer, frequently at an early age, with few known risk factors. Predictions of the response to treatment or the likelihood of developing neck or distant metastases are largely inaccurate. We still need an imaging technique that can accurately identify microscopic, nonpalpable neck metastases. Chemoradiation has too high a rate of disabling side effects. It is hoped that the advances described in the book will translate into better treatment results, sooner rather than later.

0030-6665/06/$ - see front matter © 2005 Elsevier Inc. All rights reserved.
doi:10.1016/j.otc.2005.11.006

I sincerely appreciate the opportunity to serve as Guest editor of this issue, and I thank the authors for their valuable contributions and insights. Most of all, thanks to Kathleen.

Arlen D. Meyers, MD, MBA
Department of Otolaryngology
University of Colorado Health Sciences Center
4200 East 9th Avenue
Denver, CO 80262, USA

E-mail address: Arlen.Meyers@UCHSC.edu

ELSEVIER
SAUNDERS

Otolaryngol Clin N Am
39 (2006) 229–247

OTOLARYNGOLOGIC
CLINICS
OF NORTH AMERICA

Molecular Biology of Oral Cavity Squamous Cell Carcinoma

Michael E. Kupferman, MD,
Jeffrey N. Myers, MD, PhD*

Department of Head and Neck Surgery, M. D. Anderson Cancer Center of the University of Texas, 1515 Holcombe Boulevard, Unit 441, Houston, TX 77030, USA

Oral cavity squamous cell carcinoma (OCSCC) is diagnosed in approximately 12,000 Americans and results in the death of more than 5000 each year [1]. Worldwide, OCSCC is a major health care problem, accounting for more than 274,000 newly diagnosed cancers, and is the most frequently diagnosed cancer in some regions of the world [2]. In Central and Western Europe, the mortality rates for OCSCC range from 29 to 40 per 100,000 [3]. There is also a high incidence of this disease in India and parts of Southeast Asia. Worldwide, OCSCC is the eleventh most common cancer. Although improvements have been achieved in surgical techniques, radiation therapy protocols, and chemotherapeutic regimes [4], the overall 5-year survival rate for this disease remains at 50% and has not significantly improved in the past 30 years [5].

It is now apparent that improved treatment for OCSCC hinges on understanding the underlying dysregulation of the molecular processes in OCSCC. Already, a better understanding of the fundamental mechanisms of carcinogenesis and metastasis has yielded some promising targets for treatment in various cancers [6]. Because newer diagnostic strategies and novel agents that target specific molecular pathways are increasingly being implemented in the clinical setting, it behooves the surgeon treating this disease to have a basic understanding of tumor biology. This article focuses on the current knowledge of the molecular processes that underlie tumorigenesis and metastasis in OCSCC.

* Corresponding author.
E-mail address: jmyers@mdanderson.org (J.N. Myers).

0030-6665/06/$ - see front matter © 2005 Elsevier Inc. All rights reserved.
doi:10.1016/j.otc.2005.11.003

Field cancerization and the genetic progression of oral cavity squamous cell carcinoma

The process by which a normal cell is transformed into a malignant one has been the focus of tumor biology for decades and has resulted in the description of several diverse mechanisms of carcinogenesis. Two of these, which are critical to OCSCC tumorigenesis, are field cancerization and genetic progression.

Field cancerization

Chronic exposure to tobacco and alcohol has long been associated with the development of OCSCC. Further, patients diagnosed with OCSCC who have been chronically exposed to tobacco and alcohol are at high risk for recurrences and second primary lesions. To explain the development of multiple OCSCC recurrences and second primary tumors in distinct areas of histologically normal upper aerodigestive tract mucosa, Slaughter and colleagues [7] described the phenomenon of field cancerization. It was proposed that regions of grossly normal mucosa have the following properties that increase the likelihood of transformation and recurrence:

1. Tumors in the oral cavity arise in areas of histologically dysplastic mucosa.
2. Tumors in the oral cavity are surrounded by dysplastic mucosa.
3. The coalescence of multiple small lesions results in clinically isolated lesions.
4. Local recurrences and second primaries arise from the remnant dysplastic epithelium.

It is thought that chronic exposure to environmental mutagens in tobacco and alcohol or infection with human papillomavirus (HPV) can contribute to the development of these areas of condemned mucosa. The evolution of this process is detailed here.

During the past 4 decades extensive research has been done on the mechanisms of field cancerization, and a unifying theory has begun to emerge.

Fearon and Vogelstein [8,9] were the first to describe a coherent model for the genetic basis of a human cancer, specifically colon cancer. The following four features define this model:

1. The activation of oncogenes and the inactivation of tumor suppressor genes are the results of early genetic alterations that accompany the phenotypic changes that occur in the progression from colonic adenomas to carcinomas.
2. At least four mutations are necessary for the transformation.
3. The overall accumulation of mutations, rather than the order in which they occur, is primarily responsible for carcinogenesis.
4. Alterations in tumor suppressor gene function may not require "two hits" for promoting the development of tumors.

This multistep model of tumor progression has now been observed in multiple cancers, including head and neck squamous cell carcinoma (HNSCC) [10]. The progression from normal mucosa to dysplastic epithelium and ultimately a frankly invasive squamous cell carcinoma proceeds in an orderly histologic fashion that is marked by distinct chromosomal alterations, often as the result of chronic alcohol and tobacco use.

Genetic progression

Various genetic alterations in histologically normal tissues and in premalignant lesions can be detected, including loss of heterozygosity at chromosomes 3p14 and 9p21, and these alterations are among the earliest molecular changes [11]. It is believed that these areas harbor tumor suppressor genes, and thus deletion of genes in these regions may contribute to neoplastic transformation. Mutations in the region of chromosome 17p13, which encompasses the well-studied tumor suppressor gene *p53*, are among the early events that contribute to malignant transformation [12]. Indeed, biopsies of normal mucosa from patients who have upper aerodigestive tract carcinomas frequently harbor *p53* mutations [13].

Other molecular changes that have been associated with OCSCC include the activation of telomerase activity and DNA hypermethylation. Telomerases are enzymes that maintain chromosomal length at the tips of the dividing chromosomes by adding hexanucleotide repeats to the growing complementary DNA strands [14]. Some findings suggest that the acquisition of telomerase activity occurs early in the progression of squamous cell carcinoma [15]. Another early event is DNA promoter hypermethylation, which is an epigenetic event that leads to the silencing of gene expression in CpG-rich domains. In dysplastic lesions of the oral cavity, hypermethylation of the $p16^{INK4a}$ locus, at chromosome 9p21, has frequently been observed [16].

A molecular-based update to Slaughter's original tenets has now been proposed and rests on the concept that a single epithelial cell harboring distinct genetic alterations undergoes clonal expansion, ultimately forming a region of epithelium with the potential for cancerous growth. This genetically unstable population of cells continues to enlarge, displacing the histologically similar, genetically normal mucosa. The unstable genetic makeup of this clonal population and continued exposure to mutagens from tobacco, alcohol, HPV, or all three, contribute to further "hits" resulting in malignant transformation in distinct regions of the affected mucosa (Fig. 1) [17].

Taken together, these studies provide an integrated view of how normal oral epithelium can progress, in a multistep manner, to become an invasive squamous cell carcinoma. Although a number of important questions remain to be answered, such as how specific genetic changes mechanistically contribute to carcinogenesis, it is intuitive that addressing the underlying

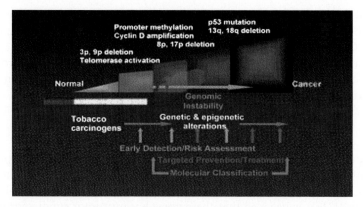

Fig. 1. Multiple alterations in the genetic makeup of epithelial cells contribute to the development of head and neck cancers. The accumulation of specific DNA mutations is required for
this process. (*From* Mao L, Hong WK, Papadimitrakopoulou VA. Focus on head and neck
cancer. Cancer Cell 2004;5(4):311–6; with permission.)

genetic insults may be a viable approach to reversing or halting the process
of malignant transformation.

Cancer-controlling genes

During the past decade, abundant research efforts have been aimed at
identifying the genes that are affected by the genomic instability that is in-
herent in tumorigenesis. Three major classes of such genes have been identified: oncogenes, tumor suppressor genes, and stability genes (Table 1) [18].

Oncogenes

Oncogenes encode proteins that demonstrate hyper-functionality in carcinogenesis and directly contribute to the malignant process. Typically,
these genes require a single allelic event to render them tumorigenic, often
as the result of chromosomal translocation, gene amplification, or a mutation. In OCSCC, these oncogenes include *EGFR* [19], *STAT3* [20], and
RAS [21], which are discussed later.

Tumor suppressor genes

Tumor suppressor genes, on the other hand, encode proteins that prevent
normal cellular processes from going awry. Cells usually require only a single
functioning copy of the tumor suppressor gene to maintain normal cellular
homeostasis. Only when a cell undergoes loss of both alleles of a tumor suppressor gene locus, through deletion, mutation, or epigenetic silencing, does
loss of cell growth control become evident. Alfred Knudson first proposed
this "two-hit hypothesis" in a study of pediatric patients suffering from retinoblastoma (RB), which has since been explained by the loss of both

Table 1
Cancer-controlling genes

Gene class	Tumor type
Oncogenes	
EGFR	Squamous cell carcinoma
Neu/c-erbB2	Breast carcinoma
RET	MEN IIA, IIB
H-ras	Colon carcinoma, lung carcinoma
N-myc	Neuroblastoma
Tumor suppressor genes	
RB1	Retinoblastoma
P53	Colon carcinoma, Li-Fraumeni syndrome
APC	Familial adenomatous polyposis
NF1	Neurofibromatosis I, neuroblastoma
NF2	Neurofibromatosis II, schwannoma
VHL	Von-Hippel-Lindau syndrome, endolymphatic sac tumor
Stability genes	
BRCA1	Breast carcinoma
XPA	Xeroderma pigmentosum
FANCA	Squamous cell carcinoma

regions of the *RB* gene, through mutation or allelic loss [22,23]. This process has since been observed for numerous other tumor suppressor genes, including *TP53* [24,25], *RB1* [26], and *PTEN* [27]. Some recent evidence, however, suggests that even genetic heterozygosity for certain tumor suppressor genes contributes to transformation. The precise mechanism for this phenomenon, termed haploinsufficiency, remains to be elucidated.

Stability genes

Genes that encode proteins that play a role in the housekeeping of the cell's DNA have been termed "stability genes." This class of genes controls processes involved in DNA-mismatch repair, nucleotide excision repair, chromosomal segregation, and the mitotic complex. These genes do not contribute directly to carcinogenesis, but when they are mutated or nonfunctional, multiple genetic insults accumulate at a higher rate. *BRCA1*, a recently described gene associated with an increased risk of breast carcinoma, is one such gene [28]. In addition, patients harboring mutations in *FANCA*, a gene that has recently been shown to play a role in the repair of double-stranded DNA breakage points [29], have a genetic predisposition to develop HNSCCs [30].

Hallmarks of carcinoma

Although the genetic changes that accompany carcinogenesis have been studied extensively, the cellular pathophysiology of tumor behavior has been elucidated only recently through the use of modern molecular biologic techniques. Although correlating global chromosomal changes with specific tumor behavior has been difficult, some basic characteristics of the typical cancer cell have been identified. In addition, although some of the mechanisms of tumorigenesis and metastasis that are innate to cancer cells have not yet been explained, an overall description of these features has been put forth in a classic paper by Hanahan and Weinberg (Fig. 2) [31]. Fundamentally, alterations in six normal physiologic processes typify the malignant phenotype of any cancer: (1) autonomy in growth signaling, (2) evasion of apoptosis, (3) unresponsiveness to growth inhibitory signaling, (4) limitless replication, (5) angiogenesis, and (6) invasion and metastasis. A brief description of each process, as it relates to OCSSC, is provided here.

Autonomy in growth signaling

To maintain cellular growth, cells harbor membrane-bound surface receptors that transduce specific extracellular signals to the intracellular machinery. The extracellular signals may arrive in the form of cytokines, growth factors, or cell–cell interactions within the extracellular space. These signals then mediate the activation of highly specific intracellular pathways, ultimately leading to cellular proliferation. Under pathologic conditions, cancer cells usurp these growth and proliferative pathways by multiple means, resulting in aberrant tumor cell multiplication. Unlike untransformed cells,

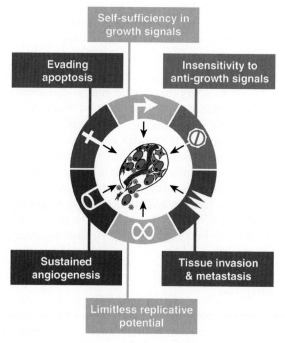

Fig. 2. Aberrant cellular processes that are characteristic of all cancers. (*From* Hanahan D, Weinberg RA. The hallmarks of cancer. Cell 2000;100(1):57–70; with permission.)

malignant cells do not require exogenous stimuli to initiate the activation of these progrowth processes; in most tumor cells, these pathways function autonomously, either through constitutive activation or autocrine and paracrine mechanisms (Fig. 3).

In OCSCC, the trait most extensively studied at the molecular level has been growth-signal autonomy. As a cancer of epithelial origin, HNSCC is marked by high levels of epidermal growth factor receptor (EGFR) activity, whose level of overexpression can portend a poorer prognosis [32,33]. The constitutive activation of EGFR through (1) expression of paracrine and autocrine epidermal growth factor, (2) gain-of-function mutations, or (3) protein overexpression is found in nearly 90% of all oral cavity and head and neck cancers [19]. Signaling through this receptor leads to the activation of multiple oncogenic and prosurvival cascades, including JAK–STAT, MAPK, PI3K–AKT, and ras [34]. The net effect of EGFR is increased downstream phosphorylation of target protein and the increased expression of the pathways involved in cell cycling, cell survival, and cellular proliferation (Fig. 4). The inhibition of EGFR-mediated signaling is thus a rational strategy for the management of OCSCC. Antibody-based and small molecule–based approaches are now in various phases of clinical development [35,36]. In fact, a recent prospective, randomized clinical trial has shown that combining the anti-EGFR antibody cetuximab (or C225) with radiotherapy for the treatment of locally advanced HNSCC leads to an overall survival benefit when compared with radiotherapy alone [37]. This finding

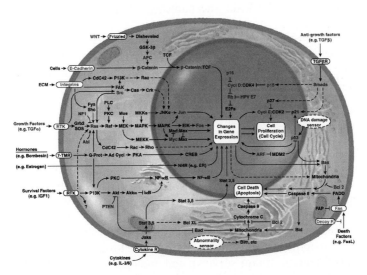

Fig. 3. An integrated map of the cellular pathways that contribute to dysregulation of cellular proliferation, apoptosis, gene expression, and DNA damage repair. Although multiple extracellular processes can be involved (eg, growth factors, cytokines, extracellular matrix proteins, and cell–cell interactions), signal transduction targets select intracellular circuits. (*From* Hanahan D, Weinberg RA. The hallmarks of cancer. Cell 2000;100(1):57–70; with permission.)

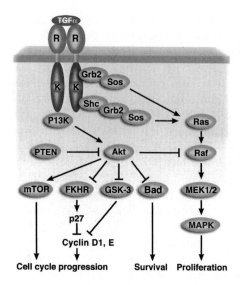

Fig. 4. The epidermal growth factor receptor activates the ras and AKT pathways through tyrosine kinase activation, leading to increased cellular proliferation, prosurvival pathways, and heightened cell cycle activity. (*From* Mendelsohn J, Baselga J. Status of epidermal growth factor receptor antagonists in the biology and treatment of cancer. J Clin Oncol 2003;21(14):2787–99; with permission.)

highlights the tremendous potential of treating OCSCC with agents that target the underlying biologic mechanisms of tumor development and progression.

One group of signaling proteins that has generated tremendous interest in the field of molecular carcinogenesis is those belonging to the signal transducer and activator of transcription (STAT) family. Initially identified as a mediator of interferon-induced cellular signaling, *STAT3* has since been shown to be an oncogene that is overexpressed in a number of solid-organ tumors [38]. Further, the level of *STAT3* expression in human tumor specimens is inversely proportional to patient survival [39]. *STAT3* has been extensively studied in OCSCC. Although *STAT3* is a downstream target of EGFR phosphorylation [40], it can also be activated by a number of upstream tyrosine kinases, including JAK, src, and platelet-derived growth factor receptor [41]. Constitutive STAT3 activity leads to the transcription and expression of a number of pro-oncogenic protein targets, including survivin, bcl-x_L, vascular endothelial growth factor (VEGF), bcl-2, and cyclin D_1. The selective overexpression of these downstream targets leads to unrestricted cellular proliferation, tumor survival, and angiogenesis (Fig. 5) [42].

Insensitivity to inhibitory growth signals

The cell cycle is controlled by multiple proteins that provide homeostatic signals that induce either cellular mitosis (M phase) or senescence (G_0

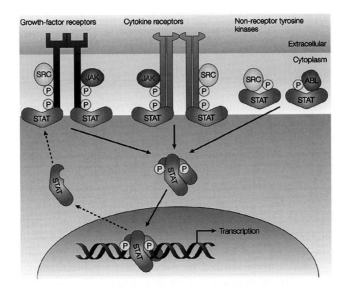

Fig. 5. STAT proteins are activated by intracellular tyrosine kinases, growth factor receptors, and cytokine receptors. Once phosphorylated, they translocate to the nucleus and initiate a specific program of gene expression that mediates prosurvival and antiapoptotic mechanisms, as well as angiogenesis. (*From* Yu H, Jove R. The STATs of cancer—new molecular targets come of age. Nat Rev Cancer 2004;4(2):97–105; with permission.)

phase). This balance between growth and maintenance is maintained by both external and internal cellular stimuli, but under tumorigenic conditions these mechanisms are shifted toward continued cellular replication by a lack of responsiveness to antigrowth signals. It is thought that alterations in RB protein function may be the primary event that allows unchecked cell cycling [26]. By interacting with transcription factors such as E2F, RB regulates the expression of genes required for DNA synthesis and replication, preventing the transition from the G_1 phase to the S phase of the cell cycle. Mechanistically, dephosphorylated RB proteins bind to the promoter regions of genes involved in replication and recruit histone deacetylases and chromatin remodeling proteins, ultimately suppressing gene expression [43]. Under pathologic conditions, the loss of *RB* or RB protein phosphorylation effectively allows the DNA replication machinery to operate unchecked.

In OCSCC, the RB system is critically important, because HPV, a proposed etiologic factor for OCSCC, can effectively inhibit RB function. The HPV DNA machinery encodes for two important proteins: E6 and E7. E6 is though to interact with *p53*, whereas the E7 protein binds to RB, leading to its degradation and the release of E2F, permitting the transcription of proproliferative genes [44]. On the other hand, the E6 HPV protein binds to *p53* and BAK, a proapoptotic protein, preventing entry into the apoptotic pathway and leading to proliferation, genomic instability, and tumor progression. Direct evidence of HPV and the E7 protein in the malignant process has yet to be demonstrated, however (Fig. 6).

Evasion of apoptosis

One of the most fundamental features of normal cellular physiology is apoptosis, or programmed cell death. This process is critically important for organogenesis, embryogenesis, and cellular homeostasis. Apoptosis can be triggered by a variety of stimuli, which can activate intrinsic or extrinsic pathways of apoptosis induction (Fig. 7) [45]. The extrinsic pathway is initiated by extracellular ligands binding to receptors such as fas or tumor necrosis factor–inducing ligand, whereas the intrinsic pathway is activated by the release of cytochrome c from the mitochondria [46]. A discrete set of proteins, termed "caspases," propagates this pathway when the death program is activated. For example, proteins encoded by the antiapoptotic *bcl* family of genes are balanced by proapoptotic proteins, including Bad and Bax. In malignant transformation this intracellular equilibrium is disturbed toward antiapoptosis and is commonly seen in OCSCC [47]. Evidence of a molecular cause for the evasion of apoptosis in human tumors was first demonstrated in follicular lymphomas and consisted of increased expression of *bcl-2* [48]. Mechanisms of apoptotic resistance in OCSCC include mutations in *p53* and *bcl-2* and its family-member proteins, overexpression of nuclear factor kappa B or AKT pathway activation [49–51]. Potential therapeutic strategies to potentiate apoptosis in tumors that target these mechanisms are currently being investigated.

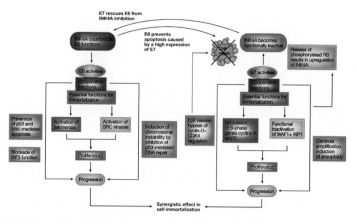

Fig. 6. HPC proteins E6 and E7 contribute to carcinogenesis by inhibiting apoptosis and inducing cell immortalization through complex mechanisms. (*From* zur Hausen H. Papillomaviruses and cancer: from basic studies to clinical application. Nat Rev Cancer 2002;2(5):342–50; with permission.)

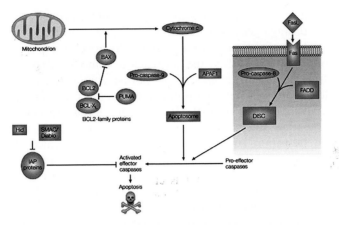

Fig. 7. Intrinsic and extrinsic pathways activate the apoptotic process. The release of cytochrome c from the mitochondria initiates the intrinsic pathway, whereas extracellular proteins binding to death receptors initiate the extrinsic pathway. (*From* Hipfner DR, Cohen SM. Connecting proliferation and apoptosis in development and disease. Nat Rev Mol Cell Bio. 2004;5(10):805–15; with permission.)

Limitless replication

Although intuitively the characteristics enumerated previously seem sufficient to account for tumor progression, other innate biologic processes take part in continued cell division. For example, transformed cells acquire the ability to undergo unlimited cycles of mitosis, a process termed "immortalization." Cell culture studies show that normal cells are able to undergo between 60 and 70 rounds of mitosis before cellular crisis occurs [52], whereby chromosomal disarray results in massive cell death. For a cancer cell to survive, it must survive this process of cellular crisis. Cancer cells use various means to survive crisis. For example, the inability of DNA polymerase to catalyze the addition of the nucleotides to the 3′ end of the chromosomal strand is believed to lead to progressive loss of the genetic code and ultimately to the aberrant chromosomal binding in these regions. One mechanism thought to abrogate telomeric loss and crisis in cancer cells is the acquisition of telomerase function. Unregulated telomeric function allows tumor cells to replicate indefinitely, whereas normal cells without telomerase ultimately senesce. Such increased telomerase activity has been demonstrated in malignant lesions of the oral cavity and is probably an early event in the progression from hyperplastic epithelium to OCSCC [15,53]. A definitive role for telomerase and its therapeutic implications have yet to be determined, however.

Angiogenesis

Although Folkman [54] first recognized the role of new blood vessel formation (angiogenesis) in human tumor progression more than 30 years ago, renewed interest in this area has spawned abundant evidence showing the importance of angiogenesis in tumor progression. The recognition during the past 15 years of the importance of tumor angiogenesis in carcinogenesis has led to a paradigm shift in the approach to tumor biology and targeted therapeutic strategies for cancers. Under normal conditions, a stable balance is carefully maintained between proangiogeneic (VEGF, fibroblast growth factors, platelet-derived growth factor) and antiangiogenic mediators (thrombospondins, interferons, endostatin, and angiostatin). At some point during the transition to the malignant phenotype, termed "angiogenic switch," tumor cells acquire the ability to sustain continued new vessel growth [55]. Only when a tumor is capable of recruiting endothelial cells to form a microvasculature can micronutrients and oxygen be delivered to the growing tumor mass (Fig. 8).

Although the mechanisms of tumor-mediated angiogenesis are currently under investigation, it is already clear that VEGF is one of the most potent mediators of this process. The endogenous expression of VEGF has been shown to be increased in various cancers and has been associated with poor prognosis and metastasis in OCSCC [56]. As one of the most potent vascular mitogens, VEGF binds to the VEGF receptor on endothelial cells, initiating signaling cascades that lead to endothelial migration, proliferation, differentiation, and increased vascular permeability. VEGF expression and differential oxygen concentrations also lead to the formation of immature, ectatic, and permeable vessels that lack pericytes and thus are different from normal small blood vessels. This difference has significant therapeutic

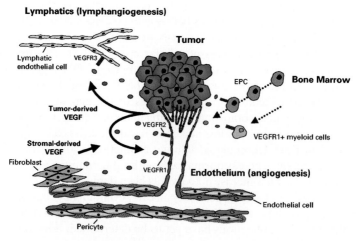

Fig. 8. VEGF protein secreted by tumor cells is a powerful mitogen, resulting in endothelial cell proliferation, migration, and vascular permeability. The various isoforms of VEGF dictate whether lymphatic or vascular endothelium will be recruited to the growing tumor. (*From* Hicklin DJ, Ellis LM. Role of the vascular endothelial growth factor pathway in tumor growth and angiogenesis. J Clin Oncol 2005;23(5):1011–27; with permission.)

implications, in that "normalizing" this vasculature may allow the delivery of chemotherapeutic agents and may sensitize these hypoxic regions in the tumors to radiation therapy [57]. Whether these findings are applicable to the complex biology in human tumors remains to be seen. Early clinical investigations in this area show promise; for example, it has been shown that bevacizumab, an antibody to VEGF, combined with irinotecan, 5-fluorouracil, and leucovorin is superior to chemotherapy alone in achieving a median and progression-free duration of survival in the treatment of patients who have metastatic colon cancer [58].

Invasion and metastasis

The hallmark feature of cancer that ultimately distinguishes it from a benign lesion is its ability to invade local tissues, spread to regional lymphatics, and metastasize to distant organs. Fundamentally, there must be a radical divergence in the tumor cell's phenotype for it to be able to survive within a new organ microenvironment. Mechanisms that contribute to this phenotype can be divided into three distinct processes: (1) alterations in cell–cell interactions, (2) degradation of the extracellular matrix, and (3) epithelial–mesenchymal transition.

The loss of normal intercellular adhesions is believed to be one of the earliest events in the process of metastasis. Cadherins, proteins that span the intercellular space between two cells, are found predominantly in cells of epithelial origin. E-cadherin, a member of this family, is a calcium-dependent protein that maintains epithelial cell adhesion and polarity [59]. Loss of E-cadherin has been shown to occur early in epithelial carcinogenesis, which correlates with the development of lymph node metastasis in OCSCC [60,61]. Cadherins are thus considered tumor suppressor genes, in that loss of expression or function leads to malignant transformation [62]. Mechanistically, cadherins initiate a program of signal transduction that suppresses growth, proliferation, and migration [63]. Potentially viable avenues for reversing the metastatic program in OCSCC include re-expression of E-cadherin or modification of its downstream signaling pathways.

Degradation of the basement membrane that supports squamous epithelium must occur for a tumor cell to invade and metastasize (Fig. 9). Matrix metalloproteinases (MMPs) are a large family of zinc-dependent enzymes that catalyze the disassembly of the extracellular matrix. MMP-9 is one of the best-described members of this family, and its expression has been implicated in invasion and metastasis for numerous tumor types, including OCSCC. Aberrant expression of MMP-9 is considered an early event in epithelial carcinogenesis and correlates with aggressive tumor behavior [64,65].

One of the most intriguing models that have been espoused to explain certain features of carcinogenesis is the epithelial–mesenchymal transition. This phenomenon was originally described in embryogenesis but is now

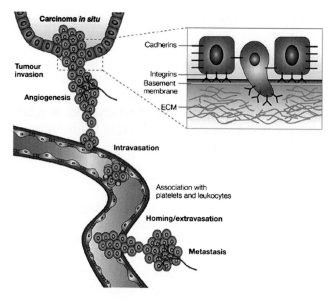

Fig. 9. Tumor metastasis is the culmination of a number of distinct processes that include basement membrane degradation, angiogenesis, detachment, intravasation, embolization, extrava-
sation, and proliferation in a new microenvironment. (*From* Guo W, Giancotti FG. Integrin
signaling during tumor progression. Nat Rev Mol Cell Biol 2004;5(10):816–26; with
permission.)

thought to play a role in tumor cell invasion and metastasis. In this process,
epithelial cells lose their apical–basal polarity, cell–cell adhesion, and cyto-
skeletal structure [66]. Once they begin to express surface proteins that characterize mesenchymal cells, they become capable of migrating through the
basement membrane and basal lamina into the extracellular space
(Fig. 10). Genes that have been implicated in regulating this process include
Twist [67], *snail*, and *E-cadherin* [68]. Although much of the biology of
epithelial–mesenchymal transition remains to be explored, progress in this
field may yield new targets for cancer treatments.

Genomics and proteomics

The advent of robotic technology and high-throughput analytical tools
has facilitated the dissection of the genetic pathways that govern tumor biology. One such analytical tool is genomics, the study of the patterns of gene
expression in a cellular system, which generally refers to the field of biology
that seeks to understand biologic processes from a global view, evaluating
all the transcriptional activity of a particular system under certain conditions. Its counterpart, proteomics, is the evaluation of the entire network
of proteins that contribute to cellular function. These two complementary
fields brought tremendous advances in the understanding of tumor biology,
primarily by allowing scientists to study the changes that occur in thousands

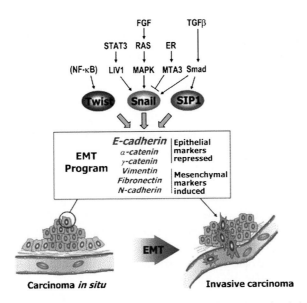

Fig. 10. Epithelial–mesenchymal transition (EMT) is a complex process that is initiated by diverse signaling pathways. The transition from a carcinoma in situ to an invasive phenotype is thought to occur through these mechanisms. (*From* Kang Y, Massague J. Epithelial-mesenchymal transitions: twist in development and metastasis. Cell 2004;118(3):277–9; with permission.)

of genes or proteins in a single experiment. Although these studies should be interpreted with care, they have contributed meaningful data to the understanding of carcinogenesis and metastasis not available by any other means. One particular tool is c-DNA microarray analysis, which has identified

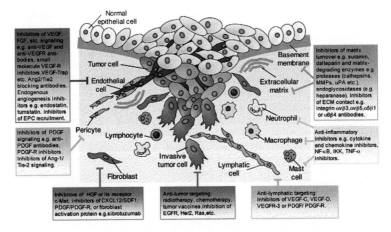

Fig. 11. Current treatment strategies have been developed to target the various compartments of the tumor microenvironment and are in various stages of preclinical and clinical testing. (*From* Joyce JA. Therapeutic targeting of the tumor microenvironment. Cancer Cell 2005;7(6):513–20; with permission.)

genomic signatures of lymphatic metastasis for OCSCC and may allow the early detection of occult metastases in select patients [69,70]. The clinical usefulness of these technologies is currently under evaluation in other tumor systems [71].

Summary

Significant advances have been made in understanding the mechanisms that contribute to carcinogenesis in OCSCC. This progress has led to the development of therapeutic strategies that target dysregulated processes in the tumor microenvironment (Fig. 11) [72]. The introduction of angiogenesis inhibitors, growth factor receptor tyrosine kinase inhibitors, and cell cycle regulators into clinical trials for the management of OCSCC has resulted from the great strides made in the understanding of tumor biology. It is important for those caring for patients who have OCSCC to have a firm background in tumor biology, because many future therapies will be based on this complex panorama of cellular physiology.

References

[1] Jemal A, Murray T, Ward E, et al. Cancer statistics, 2005. CA Cancer J Clin 2005;55:10–30.
[2] Parkin DM, Bray F, Ferlay J, et al. Global cancer statistics, 2002. CA Cancer J Clin 2005;55: 74–108.
[3] Dobrossy L. Epidemiology of head and neck cancer: magnitude of the problem. Cancer Metastasis Rev 2005;24:9–17.
[4] Cooper JS, Pajak TF, Forastiere AA, et al. Postoperative concurrent radiotherapy and chemotherapy for high-risk squamous-cell carcinoma of the head and neck. N Engl J Med 2004; 350:1937–44.
[5] Kufe DW, Holland JF, Frei E, American Cancer Society. Cancer medicine. 6th edition. Lewiston: BC Decker; 2003. p. 2.
[6] Mao L, Hong WK, Papadimitrakopoulou VA. Focus on head and neck cancer. Cancer Cell 2004;5(4):311–6.
[7] Slaughter DP, Southwick HW, Smejkal W. Field cancerization in oral stratified squamous epithelium; clinical implications of multicentric origin. Cancer 1953;6:963–8.
[8] Fearon ER, Hamilton SR, Vogelstein B. Clonal analysis of human colorectal tumors. Science 1987;238:193–7.
[9] Fearon ER, Vogelstein B. A genetic model for colorectal tumorigenesis. Cell 1990;61: 759–67.
[10] Califano J, van der Riet P, Westra W, et al. Genetic progression model for head and neck cancer: implications for field cancerization. Cancer Res 1996;56:2488–92.
[11] Mao L, Lee JS, Fan YH, et al. Frequent microsatellite alterations at chromosomes 9p21 and 3p14 in oral premalignant lesions and their value in cancer risk assessment. Nat Med 1996;2: 682–5.
[12] Boyle JO, Hakim J, Koch W, et al. The incidence of p53 mutations increases with progression of head and neck cancer. Cancer Res 1993;53:4477–80.
[13] Waridel F, Estreicher A, Bron L, et al. Field cancerisation and polyclonal p53 mutation in the upper aero-digestive tract. Oncogene 1997;14:163–9.
[14] Blackburn EH. Switching and signaling at the telomere. Cell 2001;106:661–73.

[15] Mao L, El-Naggar AK, Fan YH, et al. Telomerase activity in head and neck squamous cell carcinoma and adjacent tissues. Cancer Res 1996;56:5600–4.

[16] Kresty LA, Mallery SR, Knobloch TJ, et al. Alterations of p16(INK4a) and p14(ARF) in patients with severe oral epithelial dysplasia. Cancer Res 2002;62:5295–300.

[17] Braakhuis BJ, Tabor MP, Kummer JA, et al. A genetic explanation of Slaughter's concept of field cancerization: evidence and clinical implications. Cancer Res 2003;63:1727–30.

[18] Vogelstein B, Kinzler KW. Cancer genes and the pathways they control. Nat Med 2004;10: 789–99.

[19] Mendelsohn J, Baselga J. Status of epidermal growth factor receptor antagonists in the biology and treatment of cancer. J Clin Oncol 2003;21:2787–99.

[20] Song JI, Grandis JR. STAT signaling in head and neck cancer. Oncogene 2000;19:2489–95.

[21] Vitale-Cross L, Amornphimoltham P, Fisher G, et al. Conditional expression of K-ras in an epithelial compartment that includes the stem cells is sufficient to promote squamous cell carcinogenesis. Cancer Res 2004;64:8804–7.

[22] Knudson AG Jr. Mutation and cancer: statistical study of retinoblastoma. Proc Natl Acad Sci U S A 1971;68:820–3.

[23] Knudson AG. Cancer genetics. Am J Med Genet 2002;111:96–102.

[24] Levine AJ, Finlay CA, Hinds PW. p53 is a tumor suppressor gene. Cell 2004;116:S67–9.

[25] Vousden KH, Prives C. p53 and prognosis: new insights and further complexity. Cell 2005; 120:7–10.

[26] Sherr CJ. Principles of tumor suppression. Cell 2004;116:235–46.

[27] Shin KH, Kim JM, Rho KS, et al. Inactivation of the PTEN gene by mutation, exonic deletion, and loss of transcript in human oral squamous cell carcinomas. Int J Oncol 2002; 21:997–1001.

[28] D'Andrea AD, Grompe M. The Fanconi anaemia/BRCA pathway. Nat Rev Cancer 2003;3: 23–34.

[29] Yang YG, Herceg Z, Nakanishi K, et al. The Fanconi anemia group. A protein modulates homologous repair of DNA double-strand breaks in mammalian cells. Carcinogenesis 2005.

[30] Marsit CJ, Liu M, Nelson HH, et al. Inactivation of the Fanconi anemia/BRCA pathway in lung and oral cancers: implications for treatment and survival. Oncogene 2004;23:1000–4.

[31] Hanahan D, Weinberg RA. The hallmarks of cancer. Cell 2000;100:57–70.

[32] Rubin Grandis J, Melhem MF, et al. Levels of TGF-alpha and EGFR protein in head and neck squamous cell carcinoma and patient survival. J Natl Cancer Inst 1998;90:824–32.

[33] Xia W, Lau YK, Zhang HZ, et al. Combination of EGFR, HER-2/neu, and HER-3 is a stronger predictor for the outcome of oral squamous cell carcinoma than any individual family members. Clin Cancer Res 1999;5:4164–74.

[34] Gschwind A, Fischer OM, Ullrich A. The discovery of receptor tyrosine kinases: targets for cancer therapy. Nat Rev Cancer 2004;4:361–70.

[35] Myers JN, Holsinger FC, Bekele BN, et al. Targeted molecular therapy for oral cancer with epidermal growth factor receptor blockade: a preliminary report. Arch Otolaryngol Head Neck Surg 2002;128:875–9.

[36] Yigitbasi OG, Younes MN, Doan D, et al. Tumor cell and endothelial cell therapy of oral cancer by dual tyrosine kinase receptor blockade. Cancer Res 2004;64:7977–84.

[37] Bonner J, Giralt J, Harari P, et al. Cetuximab prolongs survival in patients with locoregionally advanced squamous cell carcinoma of head and neck: a phase III study of high dose radiation therapy with or without cetuximab. In: Proceedings of the annual meeting of the American Society of Clinical Oncology. New Orleans, LA; June 5–8, 2004. p. 5507.

[38] Yu H, Jove R. The STATs of cancer—new molecular targets come of age. Nat Rev Cancer 2004;4:97–105.

[39] Masuda M, Suzui M, Yasumatu R, et al. Constitutive activation of signal transducers and activators of transcription 3 correlates with cyclin D1 overexpression and may provide a novel prognostic marker in head and neck squamous cell carcinoma. Cancer Res 2002; 62:3351–5.

[40] Grandis JR, Drenning SD, Chakraborty A, et al. Requirement of Stat3 but not Stat1 activation for epidermal growth factor receptor-mediated cell growth in vitro. J Clin Invest 1998; 102:1385–92.

[41] Bowman T, Garcia R, Turkson J, Jove R. STATs in oncogenesis. Oncogene 2000;19: 2474–88.

[42] Grandis JR, Drenning SD, Zeng Q, et al. Constitutive activation of Stat3 signaling abrogates apoptosis in squamous cell carcinogenesis in vivo. Proc Natl Acad Sci U S A 2000;97: 4227–32.

[43] Weinberg RA. The retinoblastoma protein and cell cycle control. Cell 1995;81:323–30.

[44] zur Hausen H. Papillomaviruses and cancer: from basic studies to clinical application. Nat Rev Cancer 2002;2:342–50.

[45] Danial NN, Korsmeyer SJ. Cell death: critical control points. Cell 2004;116:205–19.

[46] Hipfner DR, Cohen SM. Connecting proliferation and apoptosis in development and disease. Nat Rev Mol Cell Biol 2004;5:805–15.

[47] Kantak SS, Kramer RH. E-cadherin regulates anchorage-independent growth and survival in oral squamous cell carcinoma cells. J Biol Chem 1998;273:16953–61.

[48] Korsmeyer SJ. Chromosomal translocations in lymphoid malignancies reveal novel proto-oncogenes. Annu Rev Immunol 1992;10:785–807.

[49] Bradley G, Irish J, MacMillan C, et al. Abnormalities of the ARF-p53 pathway in oral squamous cell carcinoma. Oncogene 2001;20:654–8.

[50] Amornphimoltham P, Sriuranpong V, Patel V, et al. Persistent activation of the Akt pathway in head and neck squamous cell carcinoma: a potential target for UCN-01. Clin Cancer Res 2004;10:4029–37.

[51] Stoll C, Baretton G, Ahrens C, et al. Prognostic significance of apoptosis and associated factors in oral squamous cell carcinoma. Virchows Arch 2000;436:102–8.

[52] Hayflick L. Mortality and immortality at the cellular level. A review. Biochemistry (Mosc) 1997;62:1180–90.

[53] Kim HR, Christensen R, Park NH, et al. Elevated expression of hTERT is associated with dysplastic cell transformation during human oral carcinogenesis in situ. Clin Cancer Res 2001;7:3079–86.

[54] Folkman J. Tumor angiogenesis: therapeutic implications. N Engl J Med 1971;285:1182–6.

[55] Hicklin DJ, Ellis LM. Role of the vascular endothelial growth factor pathway in tumor growth and angiogenesis. J Clin Oncol 2005;23:1011–27.

[56] Smith BD, Smith GL, Carter D, et al. Prognostic significance of vascular endothelial growth factor protein levels in oral and oropharyngeal squamous cell carcinoma. J Clin Oncol 2000; 18:2046–52.

[57] Winkler F, Kozin SV, Tong RT, et al. Kinetics of vascular normalization by VEGFR2 blockade governs brain tumor response to radiation: role of oxygenation, angiopoietin-1, and matrix metalloproteinases. Cancer Cell 2004;6:553–63.

[58] Hurwitz H, Fehrenbacher L, Novotny W, et al. Bevacizumab plus irinotecan, fluorouracil, and leucovorin for metastatic colorectal cancer. N Engl J Med 2004;350:2335–42.

[59] Vasioukhin V, Bauer C, Degenstein L, et al. Hyperproliferation and defects in epithelial polarity upon conditional ablation of alpha-catenin in skin. Cell 2001;104:605–17.

[60] Margulis A, Zhang W, Alt-Holland A, et al. E-cadherin suppression accelerates squamous cell carcinoma progression in three-dimensional, human tissue constructs. Cancer Res 2005;65:1783–91.

[61] Lim SC, Zhang S, Ishii G, et al. Predictive markers for late cervical metastasis in stage I and II invasive squamous cell carcinoma of the oral tongue. Clin Cancer Res 2004;10:166–72.

[62] Guo W, Giancotti FG. Integrin signalling during tumour progression. Nat Rev Mol Cell Biol 2004;5:816–26.

[63] Christofori G, Semb H. The role of the cell-adhesion molecule E-cadherin as a tumour-suppressor gene. Trends Biochem Sci 1999;24:73–6.

[64] Kupferman ME, Fini ME, Muller WJ, et al. Matrix metalloproteinase 9 promoter activity is induced coincident with invasion during tumor progression. Am J Pathol 2000;157:1777–83.

[65] Katayama A, Bandoh N, Kishibe K, et al. Expressions of matrix metalloproteinases in early-stage oral squamous cell carcinoma as predictive indicators for tumor metastases and prognosis. Clin Cancer Res 2004;10:634–40.

[66] Kang Y, Massague J. Epithelial-mesenchymal transitions: twist in development and metastasis. Cell 2004;118:277–9.

[67] Yang J, Mani SA, Donaher JL, et al. Twist, a master regulator of morphogenesis, plays an essential role in tumor metastasis. Cell 2004;117:927–39.

[68] Thiery JP. Epithelial-mesenchymal transitions in tumour progression. Nat Rev Cancer 2002; 2:442–54.

[69] O'Donnell RK, Kupferman M, Wei SJ, et al. Gene expression signature predicts lymphatic metastasis in squamous cell carcinoma of the oral cavity. Oncogene 2005;24:1244–51.

[70] Roepman P, Wessels LF, Kettelarij N, et al. An expression profile for diagnosis of lymph node metastases from primary head and neck squamous cell carcinomas. Nat Genet 2005; 37:182–6.

[71] van de Vijver MJ, He YD, van't Veer LJ, et al. A gene-expression signature as a predictor of survival in breast cancer. N Engl J Med 2002;347:1999–2009.

[72] Joyce JA. Therapeutic targeting of the tumor microenvironment. Cancer Cell 2005;7:513–20.

OTOLARYNGOLOGIC
CLINICS
OF NORTH AMERICA

Otolaryngol Clin N Am
39 (2006) 249–275

Pathology of Malignant and Premalignant Oral Epithelial Lesions

Robert O. Greer, DDS, ScD[a,b,]*

[a]*Division of Oral and Maxillofacial Pathology, University of Colorado School of Dentistry,
University of Colorado Health Sciences Center, Denver, CO, USA*
[b]*University of Colorado School of Medicine, University of Colorado
Health Sciences Center, Denver, CO, USA*

Histologic and taxonomic parameters

Oral mucous membranes and the surrounding structures are largely composed of stratified squamous epithelium that is supported by a fibrous connective tissue lamina propria and a submucosa of fibroadipose tissue. Minor salivary glands, nerves, and capillaries course abundantly throughout the supporting collagen and fibrofatty submucosa. Premalignant and malignant lesions arise most frequently from epithelium, and these epithelial lesions ultimately account for 95% of all cancers of the oral cavity. Malignant neoplasia of bone, cartilage, salivary glands, and connective tissue and those of lymphoproliferative derivatives are far less common occurrences in the oral cavity. Malignant neoplasms can and do arise from the tooth germ apparatus, but neoplasms of odontogenic elements are rare and are not included in this discussion.

Premalignant and malignant lesions of the oral mucous membrane

Erythroplakia and leukoplakia

Erythroplakia

Erythroplakia is characteristically defined as a velvety red patch that cannot be clinically or pathologically ascribed to any specific disease entity (Figs. 1 and 2). Many investigators consider erythroplakia to be the first sign of asymptomatic squamous cell carcinoma of the oral cavity [1].

* Correspondence. University of Colorado at Denver and Health Sciences Center, 13065 East 17th Avenue, Mail Stop F844, P.O. Box 6508, Aurora, CO 80045.
E-mail address: robert.greer@uchsc.edu

0030-6665/06/$ - see front matter © 2005 Elsevier Inc. All rights reserved.
doi:10.1016/j.otc.2005.11.002

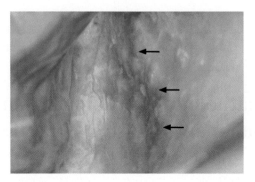

Fig. 1. Erythroplakia of the posterior buccal mucosa (*arrows*), rimmed posteriorly and superiorly by a margin of leukoplakia (Photograph courtesy of Dr. John McDowell.)

Erythroplakic and leukoplakic lesions can be considered as a continuum, because both can transition to malignant lesions. Fig. 3 shows a schematic presentation of an erythroplakic/leukoplakic continuum that defines the microscopic findings that can be seen in association with potential neoplastic change of the oral mucous membrane as the tissue progresses from benign hyperkeratosis through various stages of erythroleukoplakia.

Many systemic diseases can appear as red plaques (erythroplakic plaques), but most of these disorders have a distinctive histopathologic appearance, and they therefore are not classified as erythroplakia or leukoplakia [2]. Erythroplakic and leukoplakic lesions are sometimes categorized together as either speckled leukoplakia or speckled erythroleukoplakia; in many instances it is not possible to separate the two entities definitively.

Leukoplakia

Leukoplakia is best defined as a white patch or plaque of the oral mucous membrane that cannot be removed by vigorous scraping and cannot be classified on the basis of clinical findings or microscopic features as any specific

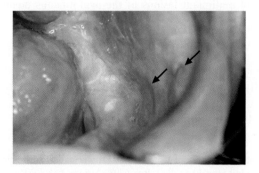

Fig. 2. Erythroplakia, (*arrows*) with a margin of leukoplakia in the buccal mucosa and retromolar trigone region. Lesions seen in Figs 1 and 2 are sometimes referred to as "speckled" erythroleukoplakia. (Photograph courtesy of Dr. John McDowell.)

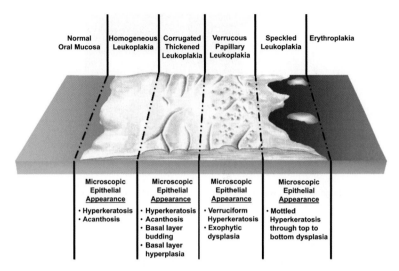

Fig. 3. Leukoplakia/erythroplakia continuum from hyperkeratosis to carcinoma in situ showing graded clinical and pathologic alterations.

disease entity [2,3]. Leukoplakia can occur at any age but seems to develop most often before the age of 40 years and with a distinct male predilection. Leukoplakia has been classified by Pindborg and colleagues [4] and by Sugar and Banocyz [5] into several different subtypes (Table 1). Pindborg and colleagues [4] have further suggested that approximately 6% of all oral leukoplakias become malignant, and Sugar and Banocyz [5] in an evaluation of 670 leukoplakic patients followed for 3 years showed that 31% of the lesions disappeared, 25% remained unchanged, and 30% improved. Burkhardt [6] has attempted to codify leukoplakia into three microscopic forms: (1) papillomatous and exophytic, (2) papillary and endocytic, and (3) plane. Most authorities, however, suggest that leukoplakia is better used as a clinical term with no distinctive histologic features that define it as a unique histologic process. Figs. 4 and 5 show examples of oral leukoplakia, with Fig. 5 demonstrating a pinpoint zone of associated erythroplakia.

Table 1
Clinical subtypes of oral leukoplakia

Authors	Leukoplakia subtype
Pindborg et al [4].	Homogeneous; white patch with a variable appearance, smooth or wrinkled; smooth areas may have small cracks or fissures, speckled or nodular: erythematous base with white patches or nodular excrescences.
Sugar and Banocyz [5]	Leukoplakia simplex: white, homogeneous keratinized lesion, slightly elevated Leukoplakia verrucosa: white, verrucous lesion with wrinkled surface Leukoplakia erosive: white lesion with erythematous areas, erosions, fissures.

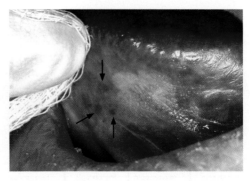

Fig. 4. Leukoplakia, ventral surface of tongue (*arrows*). (Photograph courtesy of Dr. John McDowell.)

Proliferative verrucous leukoplakia

Proliferative verrucous leukoplakia (PVL), a form of leukoplakia defined by Hansen and colleagues [7] in 1985 and more clearly defined in the past 20 years, is a series of proliferative, generally irregular white patches or plaques that progress slowly and multifocally on oral mucous membranes and in nearly 100% of cases develop into either squamous cell carcinoma or verrucous carcinoma (Fig. 6). Even when these clinical lesions are removed periodically, with apparent clear surgical margins, the lesions seem to progress. PVL is a clinically descriptive term that should not be used as a microscopic descriptor. The histopathologic corollary to PVL is the microscopic entity verrucous hyperplasia. Verrucous hyperplasia is characterized histologically by the presence of a corrugated epithelial surface that shows church-spire hyperkeratosis or so-called "toadstool" hyperkeratosis with parakeratin plugging between papillary fronds (Figs. 7 and 8) [8]. Verrucous hyperplasia can, on a microscopic level, show atypical cytologic features ranging from bland spiking hyperkeratosis to features consistent with marked severe dysplasia.

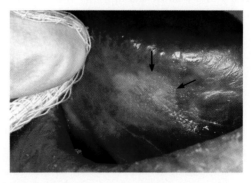

Fig. 5. Pinpoint zones of erythroplakia (*arrows*) distal to a leukoplakic plaque. (Photograph courtesy of Dr. John McDowell.)

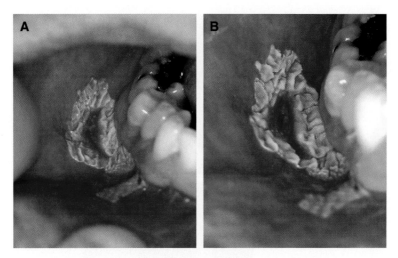

Fig. 6. (*A* and *B*) The exophytic white corrugated/papillary pattern of proliferative leukoplakia. (Photograph courtesy of Dr. John McDowell.)

The overarching clinical disease process is characterized by recurrence, persistence, and a multifocal proliferation. The progression of this process from simple hyperkeratosis to verrucous carcinoma or squamous cell carcinoma has been well documented using polymerase chain reaction (PCR) techniques. Greer and Shroyer [9,10] have also documented the presence of human papillomavirus (HPV), most frequently high-risk HPV16, -18, and occasionally -6 and −11, in PVL.

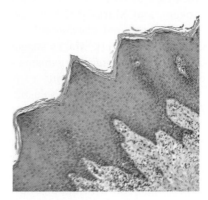

Fig. 7. Classic histologic pattern of verrucous hyperplasia with its corrugated epithelial surface and church-spire or chevron type of hyperkeratosis.

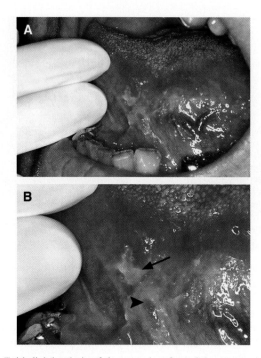

Fig. 8. (*A* and *B*) Epithelial dysplasia of the ventral surface of the tongue. Arrows in B demonstrate zones of (*long arrow*) leukoplakia and (*short arrow*) erythroplakia, which on microscopic examination were histologically consistent with moderate epithelial dysplasia. (Photograph courtesy of Dr. John McDowell.)

PVL is in fact a form of field cancerization in which tissue that appears clinically normal progresses through advanced stages of dysplasia to culminate in some form of epithelial cancer. PVL is more common in women than in men, with a peak incidence at 60 to 70 years of age. Most patients who have PVL are nonsmokers, and Marks [11] has reported that in 92% of cases he studied, the lesions harbored *Candida albicans* species at the time of microscopic tissue examination [11]. Marks suggests that it is possible that *Candida* colonization and the *Candida* organisms act as topical carcinogens in the PVL process because of their ability to produce nitrosamines, thus transforming normal oral mucosa into dysplastic tissue and ultimately malignant tissue. Typically periodic acid–Schiff stains are used to identify *Candida* organisms in PVL. This procedure is mandatory because treatment often involves surgery in association with an antifungal regimen.

Greer and colleagues [12] have reported the overexpression of telomerase, an enzyme that regulates cell longevity in cases of verrucous hyperplasia, the histologic counterpart of PVL. Some investigators have reported PVL to be an end-stage form of hypertrophic lichen planus. There is considerable debate as to whether this transition actually occurs.

Oral epithelial dysplasia

Epithelial dysplasia is premalignant condition characterized clinically by an alteration in the oral epithelium that may cause the oral mucosa to turn red, white, or some other color variation (Fig. 8). Epithelial dysplasia is characterized by atypical microscopic changes in the epithelium that can include but are not limited to prominent nucleoli, hyperchromatic nuclei, nuclear pleomorphism, altered nuclear/cytoplasmic ratios, increased atypical mitotic activity, increased individual cell characterization, basal cell hyperplasia, and basal layer budding.

Dysplasia is generally classified, microscopically, as mild, moderate, or severe (Figs. 9–11). Box 1 lists some of the atypical cytologic features diagnostic of dysplasia. Dysplastic atypia extending from the basal layer of the epithelium to include the superficial keratin layer of the epithelium is termed "carcinoma in situ" (Fig. 12). Epithelial dysplasia can become progressive over time, or, in some instances, mild forms of dysplasia may be reversible. It is unlikely that carcinoma in situ is a reversible lesion, and there is an increasing consensus among pathologists that lesions that have been classified as severe dysplasias in the past for the most part in fact represent carcinoma in situ.

Dysplasia of the oral epithelium has not undergone the close diagnostic scrutiny or extensive subclassification that dysplasia of the uterine cervix has, and the histologic classifications are still best categorized as mild, moderate, or severe. With mild dysplasia, the severity of the atypical cytologic changes is minimal. These atypical cytologic patterns become more pronounced in cases of moderate dysplasia and severe dysplasia to include altered nuclear/cytoplasmic ratios, dyskeratosis, basal layer hyperchromatism, and significant atypical mitotic forms. It has been proposed that the term "oral intraepithelial neoplasia" (OIN) be used in synchrony with the classification of the cervix and the vaginal intraepithelial neoplasia (VIN) system that is used for vaginal wall dysplasia. To date, however, pathologists have not generally accepted this proposal.

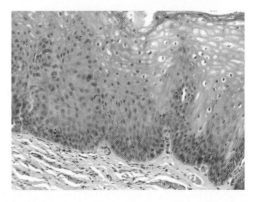

Fig. 9. Mild epithelial dysplasia demonstrating focal basal layer hyperplasia, loss of cellular polarity, and a solitary dyskeratotic cell.

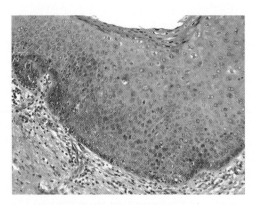

Fig. 10. Moderate epithelial dysplasia demonstrating an intact epithelial basement membrane with zones of dyskeratosis, altered nuclear cytoplasmic ratios, atypical mitoses, enlarged nuclei, and increased number of mitotic figures.

There has been significant debate as to whether dysplastic lesions of the oral mucous membrane that are in continuity with the skin surface are better characterized as actinic keratosis or as mild, moderate, or severe dysplasia. This author believes that, regardless of contiguous skin surface association, these lesions should be classified using dysplastic criteria and not simply lumped into the category of actinic change or actinic keratosis, largely because the basic biologic behavior of dysplastic lesions of the oral mucosa is significantly more aggressive than that of corresponding skin.

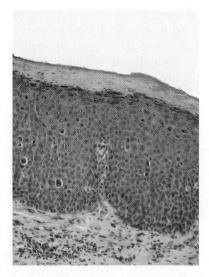

Fig. 11. Severe epithelial dysplasia with an abundance of atypical mitoses that extend high into the epithelium, zones of dyskeratosis, focal loss of cellular polarity, basal layer hyperplasia, and considerable nuclear pleomorphism.

Box 1. Common microscopic features associated with oral epithelial dysplasia

Increased nuclear/cytoplasmic ratio
Sharply angled rete processes
Loss of cellular polarity
Cellular pleomorphism
Nuclear pleomorphism
Enlarged nucleoli
Reduction of cellular cohesion
Individual spinous layer cell keratinization
Increased number of mitotic figures
Presence of mitotic figures in the superficial half of the epithelium
Basal cell layer hyperplasia
Loss of polarity of the basal cells

The risk of transformation of oral epithelial dysplasia to squamous cell cancer has been reported to be as high as 23.4%, a much higher transformation rate than the 6.5% reported for homogenous leukoplakias [1]. The anatomic location of oral epithelial dysplasia is a significant factor in assessing the risk of that dysplasia undergoing malignant transformation. Lesions of the tongue and floor of the mouth have a much greater risk of transformation than lesions at other sites in the oral cavity.

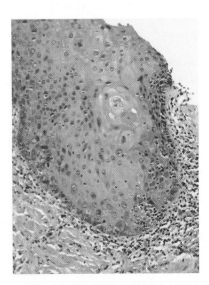

Fig. 12. Carcinoma in situ demonstrating epithelial dysplasia with marked zones of dyskeratosis. The dysplastic change extends from the basal layer of the epithelium to the fragmented surface keratin layer.

Oral epithelial dysplasia has been reported to arise in association with the vesicular bullous disease lichen planus. Greer and colleagues [13] report that 2% of 588 lichen planus cases they studied over a 20-year period underwent malignant transformation. This preneoplastic transformation is sometimes referred to as "lichenoid dysplasia," but lichenoid dysplasia is a controversial term: some authorities suggest that lichen planus does not in fact transform to dysplasia or squamous cell carcinoma over time. It has been suggested that such lesions are probably improperly diagnosed squamous cell carcinoma or dysplasia from their start. The bulk of the information in the literature, however, indicates that a small percentage of lichen planus cases do undergo dysplastic and malignant transformation.

Carcinoma in situ

Carcinoma in situ can present in the oral cavity as a red or white lesion, as some other mucosal discoloration, or as a distinct tumor mass. Mashberg and Meyers [1] suggest that suspicious red lesions in high-risk individuals have the highest propensity to develop into carcinoma in situ. The microscopic diagnosis of carcinoma in situ requires rigid histologic criteria, and the distinction between carcinoma in situ and severe epithelial dysplasia is often difficult and sometimes arbitrary. Lesions representing carcinoma in situ show a host of dysplastic changes with the key histologic feature required for the diagnosis being the presence of an intact basement membrane and top-to-bottom dysplastic epithelial dysplasia from the basal layer to the keratinized layer of the oral epithelium (Fig. 12). The characteristic features required for this diagnosis are the same as for carcinoma in situ for of the cervix.

Smokeless tobacco keratosis

In 1983 Greer and associates [14] reported a classification scheme for tissue changes associated with the use of smokeless tobacco products by teenagers and described a special form of leukoplakia, which they termed smokeless tobacco leukoplakia or smokeless tobacco hyperkeratosis. These investigators ultimately were able to identify HPV DNA in 15% of the smokeless tobacco hyperkeratoses they studied, suggesting that HPV may play a synergistic role in the development of lesions that are defined clinically as smokeless tobacco leukoplakias. In a longitudinal study in which more than 10,000 persons enrolled as high school students have been evaluated over a 20-year period, smokeless tobacco dysplasia has been a rare finding.

Smokeless tobacco is sold as either leaf tobacco or snuff, which is ground tobacco. The product, which is placed into the oral cavity, generally between the cheek and gum, contains potential carcinogens. This form of noncombustible tobacco does not result in the formation of benzopyridine epoxides seen with tobacco that is burned, and therefore the incidence of invasive squamous cell carcinoma or verrucous carcinoma does not seem to be as high in persons who use smokeless tobacco as in cigarette smokers. Smokeless tobacco products do produce a clinically identifiable form of hyperkeratosis that affects the oral mucous membrane, a hyperkeratotic plaque that is frequently referred to as a "snuff dippers patch" or "snuff dippers pouch" (Fig. 13). The lesions tend to develop directly at the site of application of the tobacco product. A similar form of hyperkeratosis has been reported in India, China, Sri Lanka, and other Asian countries in association with the use of betel nut or slake lime products. A lengthy neoplastic induction time that can range from 15 to 50 years is associated with the use of these all these products.

The histopathology of a smokeless tobacco lesion is shown in Fig. 14. A host of histologic changes can be seen in association with smokeless tobacco use, but most such lesions demonstrate hyperparakeratosis and epithelial hyperplasia. There may also be hyperplasia of the basal epithelial layer and characteristic chevron or church spire keratinization and fibrosis or scarification of an underlying collagen as well as chronic sialadenitis.

Hyperkeratoses induced by smokeless tobacco are generally reversible when the product is discontinued, but certain lesions, specifically those that have a corrugated, papillary, or velvety surface, are considered to be high-risk lesions. Shroyer and Greer [9] and Greer and Eversole [15,16] have reported that such lesions show a greater degree of epithelial atypia than lesions that have a homogeneous white surface. These investigators have also reported that more than 40% of smokeless tobacco lesions harbor HPV-specific antigens. Overexpression of the enzyme telomerase has also been reported to occur in smokeless tobacco lesions [12].

Oral submucous fibrosis

Oral submucous fibrosis is a disorder that has been reported predominately in East India, Sri Lanka, and Southeast Asian cultures. The causative agent for this precancerous lesion is thought to be related to *Areca catecha*, a component of betel nut products that is thought to affect collagen synthesis pathologically. This product, along with slake lime, is used recreationally in these geographic regions. The most common clinical presentation is thickened

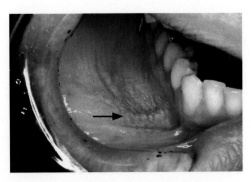

Fig. 13. Grade III smokeless tobacco keratosis (*arrow*) demonstrating a corrugated leukoplakic surface with red furrows and marked diffuseness as it extends into the buccal vestibular mucosa.

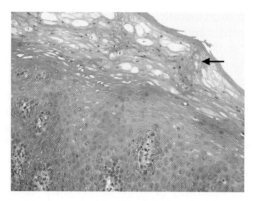

Fig. 14. Smokeless tobacco hyperkeratosis, Grade II, demonstrating chevron keratinization (*arrow*).

white mucosa lacking elasticity. Histopathologically, submucous fibrosis is characterized by connective tissue alterations in which the collagen becomes avascular and adjacent skeletal muscles atrophy. Chronic inflammatory cells may or may not be present within the collagen, and the epithelium typically shows changes that range from atrophy to hyperkeratosis. Neoplastic transformation of the overlying oral epithelium to squamous cell carcinoma occurs in some instances, as does progressive fibrosis and trismus.

Nicotine stomatitis

Nicotine stomatitis is a form of leukoplakia that occurs most commonly in the palate in patients who have been long-term smokers, most frequently pipe and cigar users. The condition seems to be proportional to the degree and frequency of the tobacco habit. In this disorder the mucosa appear white and thickened, with acanthosis and hyperkeratosis seen microscopically. Clinically, pinpoint, thin, red zones of normal oral mucosa are surrounded by circinate zones of hyperkeratosis (Fig. 15). Nicotine stomatitis

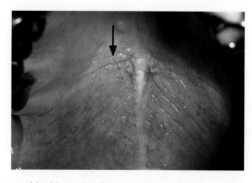

Fig. 15. Nicotine stomatitis. Note pinpoint, red, plugged minor salivary gland ducts (*arrow*) and rough textured leathery surrounding hyperkeratosis.

is easily identifiable clinically and can usually be diagnosed on the basis of a through examination and evaluation of the patient's history. Histologically, in addition to epithelial acanthosis, the lesions of nicotine stomatitis show inflammation of minor salivary glands. Salivary gland ducts may show hyperplasia and squamous metaplasia, but dysplasia is not a feature of this disorder. These red mucosal zones represent focal areas of inflammation at the point of minor salivary gland duct openings. No specific treatment is required for this condition other than to counsel patients to modify or discontinue their tobacco habit.

Malignant epithelial neoplasms

Squamous cell carcinoma of the oral cavity—clinicopathologic perspectives

A range of histologic features can be identified in squamous cell carcinoma of the oral cavity, but all show a commonality. Clinically, squamous cell carcinoma can present as a red lesion, a white lesion, an ulcer or tumor mass, or some other variation or color. Fig. 16 shows examples of oral squamous cell carcinoma.

The basement membrane of the oral epithelium is violated in all cases of squamous cell carcinoma, and the neoplastic process extends beyond the basement membrane into the connective tissue lamina propria as broad sheets, nests, cords, and islands neoplastic cells of epithelial origin. The

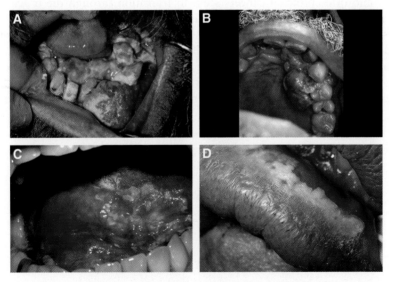

Fig. 16. (A) Exophytic squamous cell carcinoma of the mandibular alveolus. (B) Nodular hemorrhagic squamous cell carcinoma of the lingual gingival. (C) Corrugated and plaque-like squamous cell carcinoma of the ventral and lateral surface of the tongue. (D) Squamous cell carcinoma at the vermillion border of the lip.

appearance of these tumor cell nests is quite variable, depending on the degree of tumor differentiation. In some lesions, the tumor islands may show tumor cells of epithelial origin, with large amounts of keratin, mimicking the overlying epithelium. These well-differentiated neoplasms generally have minimal cellular atypia and mitotic atypia (Fig. 17). Poorly differentiated lesions, on the other hand, demonstrate little evidence of keratin formation, and atypical mitoses are prominent, as is cellular pleomorphism and nuclear atypia (Fig. 18). Th histologic appearance of moderately differentiated lesions falls somewhere between that of poorly differentiated squamous cell carcinoma and moderately differentiated tumors (Fig. 19).

Pathogenesis of oral squamous cell carcinoma

The pathogenesis of oral squamous cell carcinoma, like that of other malignancies, is related to an accumulation of multiple genetic insults that ultimately program epithelial precursor cells to develop invasive neoplastic properties. The changes that initiate oral cancer on a genetic level are related to alterations in genes that are responsible for encoding proteins that control a host of features in the development of cells, including cell motility, cell cycle regulation, cell survival, and angiogenesis. The process of clonal evolution, in which genetic mutations confer selective growth advantages on cell precursors, ultimately causing the expansion of mutant cells, seems to be the key to the multistep genetic progression toward oral epithelial cancer. Few genetic changes are required for the acquisition of a malignant phenotype, and oral epithelial cancers seem to transition through the process of aberrant cell cycle control and increased cell motility quite easily. Both of these events occur as a result of the increased expression of oncogenes and the decreased expression of so-called "tumor suppressor genes" [17]. Alterations of the groups of genes that control the cell cycle are of immense importance in the development of oral squamous cell carcinoma, and the overexpression of oncogenic proteins or lack of expression of tumor

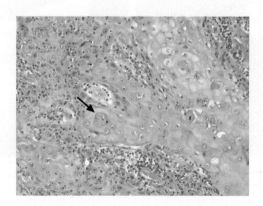

Fig. 17. Well-differentiated squamous cell carcinoma. Arrow notes keratin pearl formation.

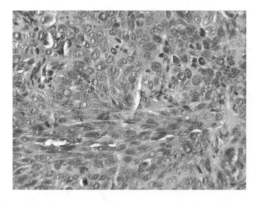

Fig. 18. Poorly differentiated squamous cell carcinoma displaying lack of keratin formation and focal spindle cell aggregation of tumor cells.

suppressor anti-oncogenic proteins can be enough to trigger neoplastic transformation. Figs. 20, 21, and 22 show schematic examples of how squamous epithelial cells also can transform to neoplastic cells through minute alterations in protein expression, cell cycle regulation, and angiogenesis.

Finally, for neoplasms to grow, they must have an adequate blood supply. Angiogenesis, the method by which this increased blood supply develops, requires the overexpression of certain tumor-induction proteins. Vascular epidermal growth factor controls tumor-mediated induction or overexpression of anti-oncogenic proteins, whereas fibroblastic growth factor and interleukin 8, a proinflammatory cytokine, are believed to be responsible in part for the promotional angiogenesis associated with oral squamous cell cancers [17].

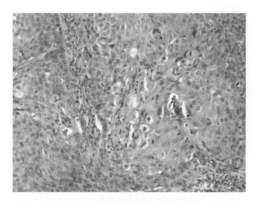

Fig. 19. Moderately differentiated squamous cell carcinoma. This moderately differentiated squamous cell carcinoma shows an accumulation of atypical cells of squamous origin with occasional nests resembling differentiated squamous epithelium and end zones of keratin formation.

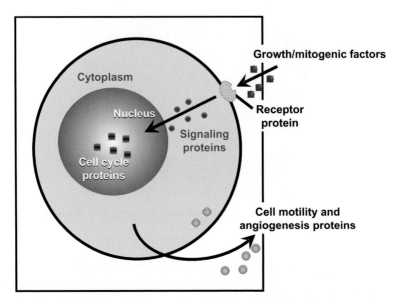

Fig. 20. Alterations in gene expression in a model of oral cancer.

Another significant factor related to development of oral epithelial cancer, especially as it relates to the replicate lifespan of tumor cells, is the overexpression or neo-expression of the enzyme telomerase. This intranuclear enzyme, present in cancer cells but absent in normal cells, seems to confer

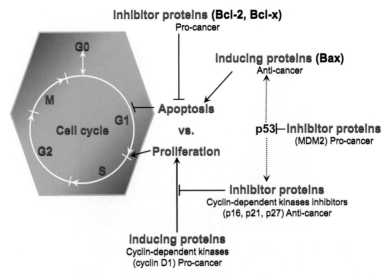

Fig. 21. Alteration in cell cycle regulation (G1-S) phase in a model of oral cancer.

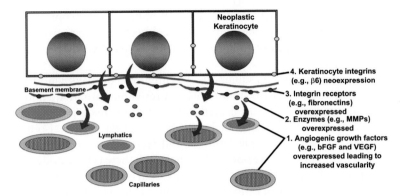

Fig. 22. Transformation of normal squamous epithelial cells to neoplastic cells through angiogenesis. bFGF, basic fibroblast growth factor; MMP, matrix metalloproteinase; VEGF, vascular endothelial growth factor.

increased longevity on tumor cells by allowing life span–controlling telomeres to retain their length at the ends of chromosomes. These telomerase–DNA protein complexes at the ends of chromosomes are responsible for cell degradation. When allowed to maintain their length indefinitely, they allow tumor cells to remain viable. Greer and colleagues [12,18] have reported the overexpression of telomerase in precancerous oral lesions.

Histopathology of oral squamous cell carcinoma

Histologically, oral squamous cell carcinomas are typically categorized as well differentiated, moderately differentiated, poorly differentiated, or undifferentiated. Undifferentiated neoplasms are often referred to as "nonkeratinizing squamous cell carcinomas." Tumors also have been classified as grades I through IV [19]. Grade I tumors greatly mimic the tissue from which they have arisen histopathologically and readily resemble their epithelial tissue of origin, where as grade IV tumors have little resemblance to oral squamous epithelium.

Well-differentiated squamous cell carcinomas are composed of neoplastic cells that have a marked similarity to the normal cells of squamous epithelium and thus demonstrate round to oval nuclei with eosinophilic cytoplasm and intracellular bridging. There may be variable degrees of nuclear hyperchromatism and mitotic activity, ranging from minimal atypia to bizarre mitoses. Keratin formation is a common feature associated with well-differentiated squamous cell carcinomas, as is individual cell keratinization. These two features are rarely seen in poorly differentiated neoplasms, and cytokeratin staining may be necessary to demonstrate these features in undifferentiated neoplasms.

The defining hallmark of squamous cell carcinoma is its invasion into the connective tissue lamina propria of the oral cavity. Thus, the classic pattern that must be identified microscopically is the infiltration of neoplastic squamous epithelial cells into the supporting connective tissue stroma. This stroma may be chronically inflamed with an abundance of plasma cells and lymphocytes.

Moderately differentiated squamous cell carcinoma displays a more varied histologic pattern in which the tumor cells may resemble normal squamous epithelial cells but with a greater degree of hyperchromatism, pleomorphism, and anisocytosis and a loss of attachment between cells. There also may be an increased frequency of atypical mitoses and decreased frequency of keratin formation. In tumors that are poorly differentiated, there is little evidence that the tumors are of squamous origin, and individual cell keratinization often is lacking. Nuclear cytoplasm ratios can be dramatically altered, and there may be significant pleomorphism among cells and considerable atypical mitoses.

Undifferentiated squamous cell carcinomas, those tumors that are commonly referred to as "nonkeratinizing squamous cell carcinoma," bear little resemblance to the tissue from which they have arisen, and defining tumor cells as epithelial in origin may be difficult. On occasion, electron microscopic evaluation may be helpful, but the more common method of identifying such undifferentiated neoplasms is immunohistochemical staining for cytokeratin using a pancytokeratin panel. Stromal changes in these undifferentiated tumors may include desmoplastic fibrosis, vascular hyperplasia, and a diffuse infiltrate of chronic inflammatory cells. The histologic grading of oral squamous cell carcinoma is subjective, and clinical staging may prove to correlate more accurately with prognosis than the grading of tumors histopathologically.

Histologic features of prognostic significance in squamous cell carcinoma

For many years pathologists have attempted to define histologic features that are of predictive value in accessing patient outcome for squamous cell carcinoma. Yamamoto and colleagues [20], and more recently Crissman and colleagues [21], have documented two significant histologic patterns for squamous cell carcinoma that may be predictive of patient outcome. These potential histologic findings include (1) the pattern of tumor invasion within the supporting collagenous stroma, and (2) the depth of tumor invasion into that supporting collagenous stroma. Yamamoto's group [20] and Crisman's team [21] reported a greater frequency of lymph node metastasis when the neoplasm's infiltrative pattern was associated with noncohesive areas of tumor cells or with the spread of individual tumor cells within the collagenous stroma.

Shingaki and colleagues [22] have reported that the depth of invasion of a squamous epithelial neoplasm into the collagenous stroma is of great prognostic significance. These authors reviewed a series of squamous cell carcinomas of the oral cavity and pharynx and were able to demonstrate that tumors that invaded the connective tissue stroma to a depth of less than 4 mm had an 8.3% rate of metastasis. Tumors that showed a 4- to

8-mm depth of invasion demonstrated metastatic rates of 35%. In tumors where the invasion of neoplastic nests was greater than 8 mm into the connective tissue stroma, the metastatic rate was 83%. These studies indicate that the depth of invasion of a squamous epithelial neoplasm into the connective tissue lamina propria of the oral cavity can be a significant factor in indicating whether metastasis will be problematic in a patient's course of therapy.

The anatomic site of presentation of a tumor can be of considerable significance in patient prognosis, and certain site-specific considerations account for variations in the behavior patterns of squamous cell carcinoma of the oral cavity. In a study of 898 squamous cell carcinomas of the oral cavity and pharynx, Shear and colleagues [23] demonstrated that tumors of equal size that involved the lip, buccal mucosa, hard palate, and the gingiva had a similar risk of metastatic spread to regional lymph nodes. The prognosis for squamous cell carcinoma arising in certain other anatomic sites, including the posterior lateral border of the tongue and the floor of the mouth, is much worse than that associated with the four aforementioned sites. Cervical lymph node metastasis, extracapsular lymph node extension, angiolymphatic invasion by the neoplasm, and perineurial invasion reflect a worse prognosis.

Investigators have made many attempts to determine the significance of positive tumor margins when there has been frozen section control of a squamous cell carcinoma at the time of surgery. Byers and colleagues [24] reviewed a series of cases of head and neck invasive squamous cell carcinomas and carcinoma in situ in which there were positive tissue margins with frozen section control and demonstrated a recurrence rate of 80% when a surgical margin was involved by tumor. Conversely, these authors found that tumors that had margins free of neoplasia had recurrence rates of 12% and 18%, respectively, for squamous cell carcinoma or carcinoma in situ.

Numerous evolving methods using an ever-increasing number of genetic and biologic markers attempt to evaluate the significance of positive tumor margins for oral squamous cell carcinoma. There have been attempts to identify the presence of certain gene products and viruses within or at the margins of oral squamous epithelial neoplasms in an effort to correlate their presence with patient outcome [25–27]. Recently investigators have attempted to use the telomerase assay as a molecular marker for identifying positive margins in oral squamous cell carcinoma when microscopic evidence of disease was not evident [28,29]. Chromosomal microsatellite markers at chromosomes 3, 8, 9, 17, and 18 and evidence of *p53* mutations in histologically normal-appearing tissue are also being used to demonstrate that genetically altered tissue which appears normal microscopically may advance to squamous cell carcinoma with certainty, given the presence of these markers [30,31].

The role of HPV in the development of oral cancer has been studied exhaustively in the past 2 decades using a host of molecular biologic techniques. More than 100 different HPV subtypes have been isolated from both benign and malignant oral mucosal neoplasms, and many investigators have identified HPV antigens and gene products in biopsies of oral cancer and oral pharyngeal cancer as well as precancer [21–23,31–35]. HPV has also been identified in normal metastasis from cancers of the oral cavity and other regions of the head and neck [23]. Recent studies have also shown that the *HPV-16 E-5* gene can induce malignant transformation of epithelial cells by enhancing growth factor–mediated intercellular signal transduction. Finally, Scully [32] has reported that oral carcinogenesis ultimately evolves because oncosuppressor genes act in cyclic association with growth factors and viruses as well as chemical carcinogens and oncogenes to initiate a process that terminates in cancer by way of the process of cyclic interdependence.

Mucosal HPVs are clearly a cause of cervical cancer and probably are the cause of a special subset of oral squamous cell carcinomas. Fourteen high-risk types of HPV have been linked to cervical cancer, and the high-risk types HPV16 and -18 have been detected with increasing frequency in head and neck squamous cell carcinoma [33].

Squamous cell carcinoma variants

Verrucous carcinoma

Verrucous carcinoma, first described by Friedell and Rosenthal [36], is a variant of squamous cell carcinoma that was fully defined by Ackerman [37] in 1948. The tumor typically appears in the sixth decade of life and accounts for 2% to 8% of all squamous cell carcinomas [37,38]. Verrucous carcinoma is best defined as a clinicopathologic process that begins as part of a histologic spectrum that germinates as a papillary verrucoleukoplakia and terminates as a malignant neoplasm [40]. Some investigators, including Shear and Pindborg [8], suggest that the term "verrucous hyperplasia" be applied to early papillary or verrucoid lesions that eventuate to verrucous carcinoma. Batsakis [38], however, has suggested that verrucous hyperplasia simply be considered an early form of verrucous carcinoma, without the necessity of a separate name designation.

Verrucous carcinoma can demonstrate multiple phases of clinical development: it can present as a lesion that can be soft and fleshy, corrugated, fibrotic, red, granular and rough, ulcerative, or papillomatous (Fig. 23) [39]. Invasive squamous cell carcinoma can be identified in verrucous carcinoma in approximately 38% of cases. These so-called "verrucoid-squamoid" hybrid lesions can be a difficult diagnostic challenge for pathologists. Therefore it is important for pathologists to section cases thought to be verrucous carcinoma thoroughly to avoid overlooking a possible squamous cell carcinoma.

A body of literature suggests that hyperkeratosis induced by the use of smokeless tobacco products predisposes patients to development of verrucous carcinoma. Shroyer and Greer [9], however, reviewed a large series

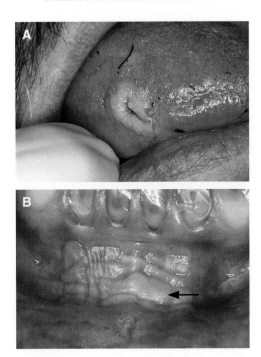

Fig. 23. (*A*) Corrugated elevated and centrally ulcerated verrucous carcinoma of the tongue. (*B*) Verrucous carcinoma of the anterior alveolar vestibular mucosa displaying a leukoplakic area of well delineated mucosal folds. Arrow denotes area of mucosal elevation. (Photographs courtesy of Dr. John McDowell.)

of smokeless tobacco leukoplakias and were unable to demonstrate dysplasia or verrucous carcinoma in any of the cases they reviewed. Their studies support the observation that smokeless tobacco use alone does not seem to initiate verrucous carcinoma in patients who had used the product for less than 7 years. These investigators, however, were able to demonstrate HPV in many of the specimens that they evaluated, and they found that 29% of 14 cases of verrucous hyperplasia that were evaluated for HPV DNA by in situ hybridization and PCR analysis were positive for HPV16. In a follow-up study these same authors reviewed 17 verrucous carcinomas and found, using similar PCR techniques, that 49% of the lesions harbored HPV16 or -11 [40]. These studies suggest that HPV may be an important cofactor in the development of verrucous carcinoma.

Grossly, verrucous carcinoma usually presents as a corrugated mass that is gray, white, or tan and is often rubbery, with finger-like or velvety projections on the surface. Microscopically the tumor is characterized by a proliferation of acanthomatous, papillary squamous epithelium that invaginates superficially as it spreads linearly along the connective tissue lamina propria displaying a broad, pushing front (Fig. 24). The surface epithelium typically shows papillary acanthosis with parakeratin plugging between papillary

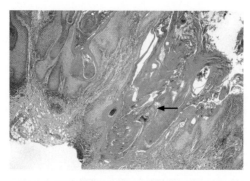

Fig. 24. Verrucous carcinoma displaying broad pushing neoplastic front, papillary acanthosis, lack of cellular atypia, and zones of interpapillary parakeratin plugging (*arrow*).

fronds, and the tumor classically demonstrates little evidence of the cytologic hallmarks of a squamous epithelial malignancy, lacking dyskeratosis, anaplasia, and atypical mitoses. The epithelial basement membrane remains intact as the tumor extends as a blunt proliferation along the connective tissue interface. Ackerman [37] suggests that this blunt proliferation of tumor along a broad, pushing front is a mandatory feature for the diagnosis of the neoplasm. Jacobson and Shear [41] have further suggested that a second highly reproducible histologic feature of verrucous carcinoma is the high incidence of a cupping margin of epithelium at the edge of the tumor that is bent or infolded on itself.

A final important feature that Shafer [42] reports is that in verrucous carcinoma a distinct wedge-like pattern of parakeratin plugging occurs between individual finger-like processes of the neoplasm. This feature is seen infrequently with other papillary lesions, such as papilloma, verruca vulgaris, condyloma acuminatum, or verruciform xanthoma, and the keratohyalin granules that are often a hallmark of verruca vulgaris and other benign papillary lesions are often lacking in verrucous carcinoma.

Differential diagnoses that should be considered when considering a diagnosis of verrucous carcinoma include oral florid papillomatous, pseudoepithelomatous hyperplasia, papillary hyperplasia, papillary squamous cell carcinoma, and keratoacanthoma. Oral florid papillomatosis is characterized clinically by multiple papillary growths as opposed to the solitary neoplastic proliferation seen with verrucous carcinoma. Additionally, oral florid papillomatosis is typically a disorder of children. Pseudoepithelomatous hyperplasia is a disorder in which the epithelial component of this reactive non-neoplastic process tends to proliferate as elongated, knife-like structures that infiltrate the connective tissue lamina propria, in contrast to the broad, pushing front seen with verrucous carcinoma. Papillary hyperplasia is easily defined clinically because of its close association with ill-fitting dentures and its typical confinement to the palate. Finally, the glassy hyalinized appearance of keratoacanthoma and the knife-edged marginal lipping that are seen with this disorder histologically are rarely seen in verrucous carcinoma.

Verrucous carcinoma can be distinguished from well-differentiated squamous cell carcinoma, with which it can be confused, by a lack of cytologic atypia and the absence of proliferation of the neoplasm beyond the basement membrane zone. Well-differentiated squamous cell carcinoma lacks the broad, pushing front of verrucous carcinoma as it invades the connective tissue and generally has no evidence of parakeratin plugging between papillary fronds.

Basaloid squamous cell carcinoma

First described by Wain and coworkers [43] in 1986, basaloid squamous cell carcinoma is an uncommon aggressive neoplasm that typically arises in the larynx. Cases have been described in the oral cavity [44,45] in sites that include the tongue base, hypopharynx, floor of mouth, buccal mucosa, and palate. Most patients who have this tumor have been smokers, and the mean age has been reported to be 62 years. The tumor has two distinct components histopathologically: (1) a component of well- or moderately differentiated squamous cell carcinoma, and (2) infiltrating basaloid-appearing nests of tumor cells. These infiltrative basaloid nests show peripheral palisading and often demonstrate central (comedo) necrosis and a high mitotic rate (Fig. 25). A spindle cell component may also be seen. The stroma between the basal cell nests can show myxoid change or hyalinosis.

The major differential diagnoses for basaloid carcinoma include adenosquamous carcinoma, mucoepidermoid carcinoma, adenoid cystic carcinoma, and small cell carcinoma. The treatment of choice for this neoplasm generally is a combination of radical surgical excision and adjunctive chemotherapy or radiotherapy. This biologically aggressive neoplasm usually demonstrates early regional and distant metastasis.

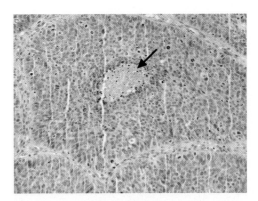

Fig. 25. Basaloid squamous cell carcinoma demonstrating central comedo necrosis (arrow) and a high mitotic rate along the peripheral margin of palisading basaloid cells.

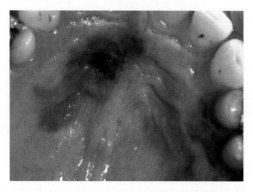

Fig. 26. Melanoma of the oral cavity demonstrating multiple dark black zones of melanoma formation, including one in the central palate and another along the lingual maxillary gingival.

Spindle cell squamous cell carcinoma

Spindle cell carcinoma has been reported in the literature under many names, including pleomorphic carcinoma, metaplastic carcinoma, sarcomatoid squamous cell carcinoma, and polypoid squamous cell carcinoma.

Most patients who develop spindle cell carcinoma are men in the sixth or seventh decade of life [46,47], and the most common site is the lip. Spindle cell carcinoma has been etiologically linked to smoking, alcohol abuse, and prior irradiation [48–50]. At present no association with HPV has found. Most spindle cell carcinomas are composed of spindle-shaped cells that are arranged in fasciae, which can be mistaken for sarcoma. When hematoxylin and eosin–stained sections demonstrate equivocal findings, immunohistochemical staining can be used to show keratin antigens.

Adenosquamous carcinoma

Adenosquamous carcinoma is a high-grade, aggressive, dimorphic variant of squamous cell carcinoma that shows both squamous carcinoma

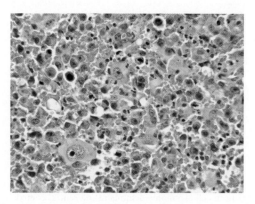

Fig. 27. Markedly anaplastic cells of malignant melanoma.

and adenocarcinoma components. The squamous component is thought to arise from the surface epithelium in the form of dysplasia, in situ carcinoma, or invasive squamous carcinoma. The adenocarcinoma component arises from the minor salivary gland ducts in the form of various grades of malignant gland formation. Gerughty and colleagues [51] first recognized this tumor in 1968. Most cases have been reported in the tongue and floor of mouth [52]. Napier and colleagues [53] have suggested that adenosquamous carcinoma may not be as rare as generally thought. These investigators also report that the volume of the adenocarcinoma component is usually significantly smaller than the squamous counterpart, rendering its recognition as a biphasic tumor difficult in many cases.

Melanoma

Malignant melanoma of the oral cavity accounts for about 1% to 8% of all melanomas. It is a rare oral neoplasm with an annual incidence of 1.2 per 10 million people. Rapini and colleagues [54] reviewed a series of 171 cases reported in the English-language literature and reported six new cases. Three of these six patients had tumors with a well-developed radial growth phase. Eighty percent of oral melanomas occur on the hard palate, alveolar mucosa, or gingiva, and the prognosis is poor, with an average survival after diagnosis no longer than 2 years.

The two principal biologic subtypes of oral melanoma are invasive melanoma, which shows a vertical growth pattern with lateral spread, and in situ melanoma, which may feature a relatively long-lasting junctional growth phase before vertical invasion. Fig. 26 shows a palatal melanoma, and Fig. 27 demonstrates the associated histopathology. A third high-risk lesion, termed "atypical melanocytic hyperplasia," although not a true melanoma, requires close long-term scrutiny by the clinician.

References

[1] Mashberg A, Meyers H. Anatomical site and size of 222 early asymptomatic oral squamous cell carcinomas: a continuing prospective study of oral cancer. II. Cancer 1976;37:2149.

[2] Pindborg JJ. World Health Organization Collaborating Center for Oral Precancerous Lesions: definition of leukoplakia and related lesions: an aid to studies on oral precancer. Oral Surg 1978;46:518–39.

[3] Silverman S Jr, Galante M. Oral cancer. 6th edition. San Francisco (CA): University of California at San Francisco Press; 1977.

[4] Pindborg JJ, Renstrup G, Poulsen HE, et al. Studies in oral leukoplakias: five clinical and histologic signs of malignancy. Acta Odontol Scand 1963;21:407–14.

[5] Sugar L, Banocyz J. Untersuchungen bei Prakanzerose der Mundschleimhaut. Dtsch Zahn Mund Kieferheilkd Zentralbl 1959;30:132–7.

[6] Burkhardt A. Der Mundhohlenkrebs und seine Vorstadien. New York: G. Fisher; 1980.

[7] Hansen JL, Olsen JA, Silverman S. Proliferative verrucous leukoplakia: a long-term study. Oral Surg 1985;60:285–90.

[8] Shear M, Pindborg JJ. Verrucous hyperplasia of the oral mucosa. Cancer 1980;46:1855–62.

[9] Shroyer KR, Greer RO. Detection of human papillomavirus DNA by in situ DNA hybridization and polymerase chain reaction in premalignant and malignant oral lesions. Oral Surg Oral Med Oral Pathol 1991;71:708–13.

[10] Greer RO, Shroyer KR, Frankhouser CA, et al. Detection of human papillomavirus in oral verrucous carcinoma by polymerase chain reaction [abstract #23]. In: Proceedings of the 49th annual meeting of the American Academy of Oral Pathology. St. Louis, MO: C.V. Mosby Co. 1993.

[11] Marks RE, Stern D. Oral and maxillofacial pathology. A rational for diagnosis and treatment. Chicago: Quintessence Publishing Co., Inc.; 2003. p. 322–6.

[12] Greer RO, Hoernig G, Shroyer KR. Telomerase expression in precancerous oral verrucous leukoplakia. Int J Oral Biol 1999;24:1–5.

[13] Greer RO, McDowell JD, Hoernig G. Oral lichen planus: a premalignant disease. Pathology Case Reviews 1999;4:28–34.

[14] Greer RO, Poulson TC. Oral changes associated with the use of smokeless tobacco by teenagers. Oral Surg 1983;56:275–84.

[15] Greer RO, Eversole LR, Poulson TC, et al. Identification of human papillomavirus DNA in smokeless tobacco-associated keratoses from juveniles, adults, and other adults using immunocytochemical and in situ DNA hybridization techniques. Gerodontics 1987;3:87–98.

[16] Greer RO, Eversole LR, Crosby LK. Detection of papillomavirus genomic DNA in oral epithelial dysplasias, oral smokeless tobacco associated leukoplakias and epithelial malignancy. J Oral Maxillofac Surg 1990;48:1201–5.

[17] Field JK. Oncogenes and tumor suppressor genes in squamous cell carcinoma of the head and neck. Eur J Cancer B Oral Oncol 1992;28B:667–76.

[18] Greer RO, Hoernig G, McDowell J. Telomerase expression in oral verrucous hyperplasia. Oral Surg Oral Med Oral Pathol 1999;88:202.

[19] Broders AD. Carcinomas of the mouth: type and degrees of malignancy. AJR Am J Roentgenol 1927;17:90–3.

[20] Yamamoto E, Miyakawa A, Kohama GI. Mode of invasion and lymph node metastasis in squamous cell carcinoma of the oral cavity. Head Neck Surg 1984;6:938–47.

[21] Crissman JD, Liu WY, Gluckman JL, et al. Prognostic value of histopathologic parameters in squamous cell carcinoma of the oropharynx. Cancer 1984;54:2995–3001.

[22] Shingaki S, Syzuki I, Nakajiima T, et al. Evaluation of histologic parameters in predicting cervical lymph node metastasis of oral and oropharyngeal carcinoma. Oral Surg 1988;66:683–8.

[23] Shear M, Hawkins DM, Farr HW. The prediction of lymph node metastasis from oral squamous cell carcinoma. Cancer 1976;37:1901–7.

[24] Byers RM, Bland KI, Borlase B, et al. The prognostic and therapeutic value of frozen section determinations in the surgical treatment of squamous cell carcinomas of the head and neck. Am J Surg 1978;136:525–8.

[25] Tanaka N, Ogi K, Odajima T. pRb/p21 protein expression in correlation with clinicopathologic findings in patients with oral squamous cell carcinoma. Caner 2001;92:2117–25.

[26] Tsai CH, Yang CH, Chou LSS. The correlation between determination of p16 gene and clinical status in oral squamous cell carcinoma. J Oral Pathol Med 2001;30:527–31.

[27] Xiz W, Lau YK, Zhang HZ. Strong correlation between c-erb B2 overexpression and overall survival in patients with oral squamous cell carcinoma. Clin Cancer Res 1997;3:3–9.

[28] Sidransky D. Nucleic-acid-based methods for the detection of cancer. Science 1997;278:1054–8.

[29] Tannapfel A, Weber A. Tumor markers in squamous cell carcinoma of the head and neck: clinical effectiveness and prognostic value. Eur Arch Otorhinolaryngol Suppl 2001;258:83–8.

[30] Vander Toorn PP, Veltman JA, Bot FJ, et al. Mapping of resection margins of oral cancer for p53 overexpression and chromosomal instability to detect residual premalignant cells. J Pathol 2001;193:66–72.

[31] Kozomara R, Jovic N, Magic Z, et al. p53 mutations and human papillomavirus infection in oral squamous cell carcinomas: correlation with overall survival. J Craniomaxillofac Surg 2005;33(5):342–8.

[32] Scully C. Oral cancer; the evidence for sexual transmission. Br Dent J 2005;199(4):203–7.

[33] Kreimer AR, Clifford GM, Boyle P, et al. Human papillomavirus types in head and neck squamous cell carcinomas worldwide: a systematic review. Cancer Epidemiol Biomarkers Prev 2005;14:467–75.

[34] Baez A, Almodovar JL, Cantor A, et al. High frequency of HPV16-associated head and neck squamous cell carcinoma in the Puerto Rican population. Head Neck 2004;26(9):778–84.

[35] Ha PK, Califano JA. The role of human papillomavirus in oral carcinogenesis. Crit Rev Oral Biol Med 2004;15(4):188–96.

[36] Friedell HL, Rosenthal LM. The etiologic role of chewing tobacco in cancer of the mouth. Report of eight cases treated by radiation. JAMA 1941;116:2130–5.

[37] Ackerman LV. Verrucous carcinoma of the oral cavity. Surgery 1948;23:670–8.

[38] Batsakis J, Hybels R, Crissman J, et al. The pathology of head and neck tumors. verrucous carcinoma. Part 15. Head Neck Surg 1982;5:29–38.

[39] Goethals P, Harrison E, Devine D. Verrucous carcinoma of the oral cavity. Am J Surg 1963; 106:845–51.

[40] Shroyer KR, Greer RO. Detection of human papillomavirus DNA in oral verrucous carcinoma by polymerase chain reaction. Mod Pathol 1993;6:669–72.

[41] Jacobson S, Shear M. Verrucous carcinoma of the mouth. J Oral Pathol 1972;1:66–75.

[42] Shafer WG. Verrucous carcinoma. Int Dent J 1972;22:451–9.

[43] Wain SL, Kier R, Vollmer KT, et al. Basaloid-squamous carcinoma of the tongue, hypopharynx, and larynx: report of 10 cases. Hum Pathol 1986;17:1155–66.

[44] Coletta R, Cotrim P, Almeida O, et al. Basaloid squamous carcinoma of the oral cavity: a histologic and immunohistochemical study. Oral Oncol 2002;38(7):723.

[45] Raslan W, Barnes L, Krause J, et al. Basaloid squamous cell carcinoma of the head and neck: a clinicopathologic and flow cytometric study of 10 cases with a review of the literature. Am J Otolaryngol 1994;15:204–11.

[46] Zarbo R, Crissman J, Venkat H, et al. Spindle cell carcinoma of the upper aerodigestive tract mucosa. An immunohistologic and ultrastructural study of 18 biphasic tumors. Am J Surg Pathol 1986;10:731–53.

[47] Goellner J, Devine D, Weiland L. Pseudosarcoma of the larynx. Am J Clin Pathol 1973;59: 312–26.

[48] Larsen E, Duggan M, Inque M. Absence of human papilloma virus DNA in oropharyngeal spindle cell squamous carcinoma. Am J Clin Pathol 1994;101:514–8.

[49] Ellis G, Corio RL. Spindle cell carcinoma of the oral cavity. A clinicopathologic study of 59 cases. Oral Surg Oral Med Oral Pathol 1980;50:522–34.

[50] Wharton J, Boguniewicz A, Jennings T. Sarcomatoid tumors of the upper respiratory tract after irradiation: a comparative study [abstract]. Am J Clin Pathol 1994;102:525.

[51] Gerughty R, Henninger Brown F. Adenosquamous carcinoma of the oral, nasal, and laryngeal cavities. A clinicoathologic survey of ten cases. Cancer 1968;22:1140–54.

[52] Scully C, Porter S, Speight P, et al. Adenosquamous carcinoma of the mouth: a rare variant of squamous cell carcinoma. J Maxillofac Surg 1999;28(2):125–8.

[53] Napier S, Gormely J, Newlands C, et al. Adenosquamous carcinoma. A rare neoplasm with an aggressive course. Oral Surg Oral Med Oral Pathol 1995;79(5):607–11.

[54] Rapini RP, Golitz LE, Greer RO Jr, et al. Primary malignant melanoma of the oral cavity. A review of 177 cases. Cancer 1985;55:1543–51.

OTOLARYNGOLOGIC
CLINICS
OF NORTH AMERICA

ELSEVIER
SAUNDERS

Otolaryngol Clin N Am
39 (2006) 277–294

An Overview of Epidemiology and Common Risk Factors for Oral Squamous Cell Carcinoma

John D. McDowell, DDS, MS[a,b,*]

[a]Department of Diagnostic and Biological Sciences, Division of Oral Diagnosis, Oral Medicine
and Forensic Sciences, University of Colorado School of Dentistry, Mail Stop F844,
PO Box 6508 Aurora, CO 80045 USA
[b]Mountain-Plains AIDS Education and Training Center, University of Colorado School of
Medicine, Denver, CO, USA

Currently available data indicate that approximately one in three Americans develops a malignancy in their lifetime. The chances of developing a malignancy increase with age and several contributing risk factors to include use of tobacco and alcohol. Notwithstanding significant decreases in death rates from heart disease, cerebrovascular disease and infections over the previous 50 years, for many forms of cancer, death rates remain essentially unchanged during that same time period. Age-adjusted data presently available through the Centers for Disease Control and Prevention, National Cancer Institute, and the North American Association of Central Cancer Registries indicate that during 2001 there were nearly 500 new cancers per 100,000 individuals in the United States. The American Cancer Society and the National Cancer Institute's Surveillance, Epidemiology and End Results (SEER) report indicates that of these new cancer cases, approximately 5% were cancers involving the oral cavity or adjacent structures. Although this rate for oral cancer indicates that oral cancers are not common, oral cancers certainly are not rare. The most recent data combined from broad geographic areas indicate that oral cancer represents approximately 3% of all newly-reported cancers in the United States. Best estimates indicate that approximately 30,000 new cases of oral and pharyngeal cancer (OPC) will be diagnosed in 2005. Despite significant advances in the treatment of other cancers, morbidity and mortality associated with oral cancer

* Division of Oral Diagnosis and Oral Medicine, University of Colorado School of
Dentistry Mail Stop F844, PO Box 6508 Aurora, CO 80045.
   E-mail address: john.mcdowell@uchsc.edu

0030-6665/06/$ - see front matter © 2005 Elsevier Inc. All rights reserved.
doi:10.1016/j.otc.2005.11.012   *oto.theclinics.com*

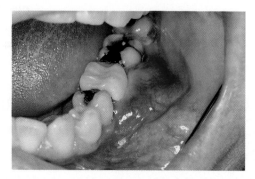

Fig. 1. Metastatic breast cancer (to right mandible) involving buccal vestibule.

remains high. The long term prognosis for OPC is much improved when the lesion is discovered early in its course. Because so many patients with OPC will be diagnosed late in their disease, only half of these new cases will be alive 5 years from the time of diagnosis. Prevention and early diagnosis remain the best instruments in our armamentarium for reducing the death and disability rates associated with oral cancers.

An oral malignancy may be primary to the mouth, metastatic from a distant site to the jaws or adjacent structures (ie, breast or lung) [Fig. 1] (metastatic breast cancer) or an oral manifestation of a lesion progressing intraorally from a primary lesion in an adjacent structure like the maxillary sinus or nasal cavity. Because more than 90% of primary oral malignancies are carcinomas, the emphasis of this article will be on the most common of the oral carcinomas, squamous cell carcinoma.

Oral mucosal squamous cell originates in the basal cell layer of the oral mucosa. The typical presentation for an oral mucosal squamous cell carcinoma is most commonly a symptomatic or asymptomatic superficial ulcer. These superficial ulcers often progress into a symptomatic or asymptomatic exophytic nodule or tumor with an eroded/ulcerated surface [Figs. 2 and 3].

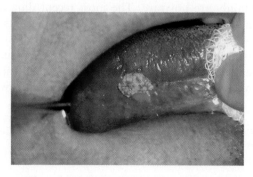

Fig. 2. Squamous cell carcinoma (right lateral tongue, 59-year-old Caucasian male).

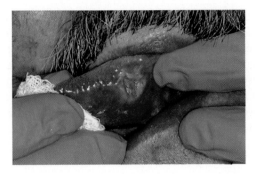

Fig. 3. Squamous cell carcinoma (left lateral tongue, 48-year-old Caucasian male with AIDS diagnosis).

Most oral mucosal squamous cell carcinomas begin as superficial ulceration progressing to direct invasion of the deeper structures resulting in a firm, nonmovable mass.

Incidence, prevalence, and death rate

Over the previous 50 years, early diagnosis and appropriate medical treatments have resulted in significant decreases in death rates from heart diseases, cerebrovascular diseases, and respiratory diseases. Some forms of cancers, particularly leukemias and lymphomas, have had significant decreases in the death rates during this time period. Although cancer of the lung and bronchus remain the most commonly diagnosed non-skin cancer in the United States, deaths directly related to lung cancer also have decreased during the time period from 1990 to 2000. Death rates from colon/rectum, prostate and stomach also have decreased during the time period from 1995 to 2000. Notwithstanding these and other advances in cancer treatment and trends toward a slight decrease in the incidence of oral cancer, American death rates from oral cancers have remained essentially unchanged since the 1960s.

Present data available through the American Cancer Society indicate that in 2005 an estimated 30,000 Americans will be newly diagnosed with cancers of the mouth or oropharynx. Unfortunately, only about half of the individuals diagnosed with oral cancer will be alive 5 years following their diagnosis. Each year, approximately 7000 Americans die because of oral and pharyngeal cancer with the median age at death from cancer of the oral cavity reported to be 68 years of age [1–4].

For descriptive purposes, most investigators separate into finite categories individual factors or conditions increasing the risk for oral cancers. Increased oral and pharyngeal cancer rates have been reported for many factors, including tobacco and alcohol use, viral infections, candidal infections, immune status, genetics, marital status, sexual activities, occupational exposures, systemic disease, dental health, socioeconomic status, nutrition, meat consumption, and a number of different lifestyles. Although one risk category often cannot be separated completely from the others (ie, alcohol and tobacco use), the categories listed below can help the reader understand a patient's relative risk for developing a primary malignancy of the oral cavity. However, it must be emphasized that oral cancer can occur with or without these relative risk factors in any person and that oral cancer screenings should be performed on every patient.

Risk factors for developing oral cancer

No single factor causes an oral cancer. Oral squamous cell carcinoma is most likely caused by a combination of extrinsic and intrinsic factors acting in concert over a (long) period of time. Indications exist demonstrating that there is at least a contributing component related to a genetic susceptibility of the individual exposed to carcinogens and a potential for malignant transformation of the oral/pharyngeal tissues. Discussing the potential genetic component increasing an individual's risk for oral cancer is beyond the scope of this article.

Over the last decade there has been significant progress made in determining the complex role that viruses play in malignant transformation. Although a brief discussion of the role that a small number of viruses play in developing an oral malignancy is included, in addition to a discussion of cellular genetics, that material can be best acquired through an extensive literature review of basic scientists and clinicians working within that field of research. The clinician should know that through the influence of viruses, changes can occur in genes that encode for the cell cycle, cell survival, and angiogenesis and that a small number of these genetic changes can result in acquisition of the malignant phenotype. This influence is especially true when there is a lack of normal immunosurveillance as is seen in HIV infections.

Epidemiologic data indicate that a strong correlation exists between exposure to many potential carcinogens and the increased risk for development of an oral cancer following long exposure or early exposure to these carcinogens. Many studies have shown that several factors lead to an increase in the relative incidence of oral cancer. Most published reports indicate that age, gender, race, tobacco use, alcohol use (especially tobacco and alcohol in combination), presence of a synchronous cancer of the upper aerodigestive track, poor nutritional status, infection with certain viruses, oral lichen planus, and immune deficiencies all increase the relative risk for developing an oral cancer. Exposure to some of these extrinsic risk factors varies significantly between ethnic groups and geographic locations globally and regionally.

The incidence of oral cancer is low in most Western countries when compared with many developing countries, whereas oral cancer is one of the most common cancers in other parts of the world. In these developing countries, oral cancer may affect younger men and younger women more frequently than seen in the United States. In northern France, the Indian subcontinent, and other parts of Asia, the oral cancer incidence rates are significantly higher than in the United States [5–7]. Reports of decreasing oral cancer trends exist in some developed countries, whereas a world-wide increase has occurred in the incidence of oral cancer [7–16]. Additionally, reported trends have occurred indicating oral malignancies appearing at an earlier age with the number of cases in women rapidly approaching the number of cases in men [7–16].

Health care providers that treat diseases of the oral cavity and oropharynx should be familiar with the common risk factors for oral/pharyngeal malignancies. Some of the most common risk factors are described in the following text.

Age and gender

Increasing age has been described as a risk factor for many forms of cancer. Increasing age allows for longer exposure to potential carcinogens and for potential damage to the DNA of these aging cells. Oral and pharyngeal cancer rates increase with increasing age with more than half of all OPC diagnosed in individuals over the age of 65. According to the National Cancer Institute SEER Program, the median age of diagnosis for OPC is 63 with the lifetime probability of developing an oral cancer being 1 in 72 [1]. Consistent with these data, most investigators report that about 90% of oral cancers occur in individuals over 40 years of age with 65 as the average age at diagnosis [1–4,17]. However, this picture may be changing in the United States and other countries. Several investigators have reported an increase in oral cancers diagnosed in younger patients [18–21] further sensitizing clinicians to the need to screen all patients for oral cancer.

Health care providers should be aware of these age-related rates for oral cancer. Patients under the age of 20 represent approximately 0.8% of oral cancer diagnoses, about 3% of oral cancers were discovered in patients between 20 and 34; 8% were found in patients between 35 and 44; 20% between the ages 45 and 54; 23% between ages 55 and 64; 23% between 65 and 74; 17% between 75 and 84; and 5.8% in patients 85 years of age and older [1].

Men are more likely to develop a malignancy than are women. As reported in the 13 SEER geographic areas for the time period from 1998 to 2002 [1], the overall age-adjusted incidence rate for all cancers was 469.7 per 100,000 men and women per year. For white men the age-adjusted incidence rate was 556.4 per 100,000 white men; for white women it was 429.3 per 100,000 white women; for black men it was 682.6 per 100,000 black men; and for black women it was 398.5 per 100,000 black women [1]. For the

SEER areas, incidence rate for oral cancer is between two and four times higher for men than women for all racial/ethnic groups except for Filipinos where the rates are similar for the two genders [1]. The incidence rates reported for Americans are not inconsistent with the rest of the developed countries [11–14,22].

Other studies have shown that trends oral cancer rates in women are approaching those rates found in men. A retrospective study conducted in the Netherlands reviewing the records of over 300 women diagnosed with oral squamous cell carcinomas indicated that rates closely approximated those of men [23]. This same study also found that the women patients presenting with oropharyngeal cancers were younger and had a higher incidence of smoking and a positive history of heavy drinking [23].

Additionally, men are more likely to die from cancer than are women of the same age. According to the American Cancer Society's SEER study [1], the age-adjusted death rate for the period from 1998 to 2002 for white men was 242.5 per 100,000 white men; for white women, it was 164.5 per 100,000 white women; for black men, it was 339.4 per 100,000 black men; and for black women it was 194.3 per 100,000 black women [1]. The age-adjusted death rate for white women is less than half that of white men (1.6:3.9 per 100,000) [1].

Race

Oral cancer is found in all racial/ethnic groups with some groups consistently reported to be at higher risk for developing these malignancies. However, reported differences in rates among racial/ethnic populations should be interpreted with caution. Asian/Pacific Islander and Hispanic figures might be underestimated because of differences in registry operations or racial misclassifications. In some countries, oral cancer is the most common form of malignancy far exceeding the incidence of other cancers. When compared with the United States, higher rates of oral cancer have been reported in India, Southeast Asia, Hungary, and northern France. Lower OPC incidence rates are reportedly found in Mexico and Japan. Whereas there might be racial/ethnic differences in cancer rates, increased oral cancer rates often are related to environmental and lifestyle choices.

The most recent SEER report indicated that blacks have higher incidence rates for many forms of cancer, including larynx; prostate; stomach; myeloma; oral cavity and pharynx; esophagus; liver; pancreas; lung and bronchus; pancreas; small intestine; and colon, rectum, and bladder [1]. Before age 55, oral cancer is the sixth most common cancer in white men but is the fourth most common cancer in black men. The SEER report also indicates that for men, the highest rates for oral cancer are found in blacks followed by non-Hispanic whites/whites, Vietnamese-Americans and native Hawaiians [1]. For several racial/ethnic groups, the number of cases are too few to reliably state the incidence rates.

In some states oral cancer rates in black Americans approaches 25 per 100,000. Black/white incidence rate ratios exceed two for cancers of the oropharynx, tonsil, and palate. Lip and salivary gland tumors are the only two types of oral/perioral cancers lower among black Americans than those rates found in white Americans.

These figures may not hold for recent immigrants to the United States irrespective of racial/ethnic group. As more Asians immigrate to the United States bringing with them social habits from their country of origin (including habits to include reverse tobacco smoking, use of areca [betel] nut mixed with tobacco, slaked lime and spices), it is expected that oral cancer rates will increase. Physicians and dentists should counsel patients found to be participating in the behaviors placing their patients at increased risk for oral cancer.

Racial/ethnic differences are not limited to incidence rates. A significant disparity continues to exist between racial/ethnic group survival rates for Americans diagnosed with oral cancer. The 5-year survival rate following diagnosis of an oral cancer is approximately 60% in white Americans. The 5-year survival rate for is only 36% for black Americans [1]. A significant part of the problem is likely to be related to poor access to oral health care for American blacks and, therefore, diagnosis in late stage of disease.

Presence of other upper aerodigestive track cancers

When a cancer of the upper aerodigestive track is found, it is important to assess the patient for the presence of another primary malignancy of the associated structures. Several researchers have reported that patients with an OPC have a greater risk for a synchronous (different site within 6 months) or metachronous (different site after 6 months or same site after 3 years) malignancy of the upper aerodigestive track. Day and Blot reported that patients with a primary OPC were at risk for developing a second cancer of the mouth or pharynx and were at a high risk for developing a primary respiratory cancer [24]. Increased risks also were reported for cancers diagnosed 5 years or more after the oral cancer suggesting that the second cancers were new primary cancers and not misdiagnosed metastases.

The increased risk for a second cancer is not limited to a cancer developing in the directly appertaining structures. The risk for developing esophageal cancer is significantly higher in men with a previously diagnosed head and neck cancer, especially if the primary tumor was located on the floor of the mouth or the pharynx [25–27].

Increased risk for a second cancer continues throughout the life of the patient. These increased risks are found in men and women and black and white patients and was most pronounced among patients younger than 60 years of age [24]. Because of the increased risk for developing a synchronous or metachronous malignancy following the initial diagnosis of an OPC, patients should be counseled regarding the increased risk for a second cancer, especially if the patient continues to use alcohol and tobacco.

Tobacco

The World Health Organization estimates that, worldwide, 1 billion people smoke cigarettes on a regular basis. Of those smokers, approximately 4 million people die every year with the number of deaths expected to increase every year unless the prevalence of smoking decreases. Most of those deaths are from heart disease, respiratory disease, strokes, upper aerodigestive track cancers, and other cancers directly related to the use of cigarettes. Cigarette smoking also causes disabilities resulting in reduction in the quality of life for an additional 10 to 20 million people.

Smoking tobacco has long been implicated in the development of cancers in many different organ systems, including all components of the upper aerodigestive track. A strong correlation of cigarette smoking exists to cancers of the bladder, kidney, pancreas, and cervix. Additionally, cigarette smoking may be related to an increased risk for acute myeloid leukemia. Depending on the product, tobacco may contain in excess of 50 established or potential carcinogens that may increase relative risks for cancers by differing mechanisms, including causing mutations that disrupt cell cycle regulation or through an effect on the immune system.

Since 1965, cigarette smoking has decreased in the United States. With this decreased cigarette smoking among men, death rates for men from lung cancer have declined slowly but steadily since 1985. Unfortunately, death rates in women did not begin to decline until the late 1990s.

The Centers for Disease Control and Prevention Tobacco Information and Prevention Sources reported [28] these data on youth:

- 28.4% of high school students in the United States are current cigarette smokers with slightly more boys than girls reporting that they currently smoke cigarettes.
- 10.1% of middle schools students in the United States are current cigarette smokers with equal numbers of boys and girls reporting currently smoking cigarettes.
- 10.4% of whites, 9.4% of African-Americans, 9.1% of Hispanics and 7.4% of Asian-Americans in middle school are current cigarette smokers.
- Each day, nearly 4400 young people between the age of 12 and 17 initiate cigarette smoking in the United States.

These figures for smoking among younger persons are especially alarming because beginning smoking at a younger age increases the risk for developing an oral mucosal squamous cell carcinoma. Marx and Stern [29] have reported that the pack-year history is less predictive of risk for oral cancer than is the combination of pack-years and age at which cigarette smoking began. Although a decrease occurred in tobacco use by high school students in the most recent reporting period, it is still worrisome that cigarette use among high school students between 2000 and 2002 was 22.9%, cigar use was 11.6%, bidi use was 2.6%, and kretek use was 2.7% [28]. Unfortunately, no significant decrease occurred in tobacco usage among middle school students during that same time period [28].

Bidi smoking is another significant risk factor for developing upper aerodigestive track disease, oral mucosal squamous cell carcinoma, lung cancer, stomach cancer, and esophageal cancer [30–32]. Bidis, flavored or unflavored, are small, hand-rolled cigarettes that consist of tobacco wrapped in tendu or temburni leaf. Bidis are imported to the United States from India and other Asian countries and have become somewhat popular among teenagers in the United States [33,34]. Using a convenience sample, Massachusetts' teenagers were questioned why they smoke bidis instead of cigarettes. The most common responses from the questioned teenagers included bidis tasted better (23%), were cheaper (18%), were safer (13%) and were easier to buy (12%) [35]. All persons, especially young persons, should be counseled that there is no safe tobacco product and that with continued use of bidis an increased risk for developing an oral cancer above that which is found in nonsmokers exists.

Kreteks are an Indonesian cigarette product that is being imported to the United States. Kreteks are clove-infused tobacco cigarettes usually wrapped in an ironed cornhusk or cigarette paper. Kreteks may or may not have flavoring agents or spices added with the other components of these "clove cigarettes." Kreteks have been shown to have higher concentrations of nicotine, tar, and carbon dioxide than conventional cigarettes [33]. An estimated 2.7% of high school students are current kretek smokers [35–37]. Although no research studies have been performed in the United States on the long-term health effects of kreteks, Indonesian research has shown that regular kretek smokers have a significantly higher risk for abnormal lung function when compared with nonsmokers [38]. Smoking kreteks is also reported to increase the relative risk for developing lung injury (especially among susceptible individuals with asthma or respiratory infections) [39]. Although it seems that kretek usage is not increasing among American teenagers, any exposure to tobacco or products containing tobacco at an early age is of great concern.

Cigar and pipe smoking also has been shown to increase the relative risk for developing an upper aerodigestive track disease, cancer of the pancreas, and significantly increases the relative risk for developing an oral cancer [40,41].

The greatest risk for several forms of oral mucosal squamous cell carcinomas is found with a peculiar habit of "reverse" smoking (keeping the lit end of the cigar or cigarette in the mouth). This form of smoking is not common in the United States but frequently is found in India, southeastern Asia, some parts of Africa, and central and South America. A significant relative risk seems to exist in cancers of the palate (an uncommon site for squamous cell carcinoma) in reverse smokers. With immigration to the United States from these countries, clinicians may see more patients with palatal cancers.

Chewing tobacco and snuff

Spit tobacco is a type of tobacco that is placed inside the mouth and has been called "smokeless tobacco." Spit tobacco is made from a mixture of tobacco and other substances to include sweeteners, abrasives, salts, and other chemical substances. While in the mouth, the product gives the user a constant exposure to the substances released when exposed to saliva. Spit tobacco commonly is used in one of three forms. "Chew" is a leafy form of the tobacco usually sold in pouches. "Plug" is chew tobacco that has been compressed into a brick form. "Snuff" is a powdered form of tobacco (described as "wet" or "dry") usually sold in tins or flat cans. In any of its forms, spit tobacco usually is placed in the mouth between the cheek and gums. Depending on the type of smokeless tobacco used, these products contain varying amounts of known carcinogens, including those compounds known to increase risk for oral/pharyngeal cancers.

Although many organizations have reported that an increased risk for oral and pharyngeal cancer exists when smokeless tobacco is used, there has been some debate as to whether smokeless tobacco (when other risk factors for cancer are removed) is a direct cause of oral cancers. Based on data collected from a number of different sources, Marx and Stern have written that smokeless tobacco products "are not significantly carcinogenic and, despite the claims of several organizations, do not produce a higher incidence of oral squamous cell carcinoma than that which spontaneously occurs in the nonsmoking, nonusers of smokeless tobacco population" [41]. Marx and Stern also present evidence from reviews of oral pathology files in Texas, Colorado, and North Carolina to show that there is no increased rate of verrucous or invasive squamous cell carcinoma related to smokeless tobacco and that they therefore can document that increased risk for oral cancer with smokeless tobacco use is "coincidental rather than causative." [41] At least one other American study seems to confirm this claim. Bouquot and Meckstroth studied the state with the highest per capita smokeless tobacco usage, West Virginia, and found that West Virginia had less oral/pharyngeal cancer than the United States average [42]. Other reports have also indicated that there is no increased risk for cancer associated with smokeless tobacco use [43,44].

A 1981 study in North Carolina indicated that there was a significant increase in oral cancers in women snuff users, especially for tissues in direct contact with the tobacco [45]. This study has been used repeatedly to support the premise that the relative rates for oral cancer are increased when smokeless tobacco is used. Other subsequent studies and reports have indicated an increased relative risk for developing an oral cancer when using smokeless tobacco [46–49].

It is the author's opinion that no tobacco or tobacco-containing product should be considered "safe" or "risk-free," especially if it is smoked. Further, a strong correlation seems to exist between relative incidence rates for oral cancer and the age at which tobacco use begins, the amount of tobacco used, how the tobacco is used, and whether tobacco use is combined with other risk factors (ie, alcohol).

Alcohol

Alcohol abuse, especially when combined with tobacco in any form, is a significant factor in the development of oral cancers [50–56]. Attributable risk estimates indicate that tobacco smoking and alcohol account for approximately three fourths of all oral and pharyngeal cancers in the United States. Alcohol abuse seems to be the second largest risk factor (after smoking tobacco) for developing an oral/pharyngeal cancer. A strong correlation exists between excessive alcohol consumption, cirrhosis of the liver, and oral/pharyngeal cancers [52]. Nutritional deficiencies associated with heavy alcohol consumption also increase the relative risk for developing an oral/pharyngeal cancer. An association with oral cancer and alcohol-based mouth rinses has not been established.

Trends in the developed countries show that oral cancer seems to be correlated closely with changes in alcohol consumption [57,58]. A strong dose-dependent association also exists between relative risk for oral/pharyngeal cancer and alcohol consumption with the risk for developing a cancer [50–59]. Unfortunately, the risk for oral/pharyngeal cancer also persists for several years after cessation of drinking alcohol [59].

The relationship between oral cancer and alcohol consumption seems to be independent of the type of alcohol consumed and is associated more directly with the amount of ethanol consumed and the length of time that alcohol has been used. Because of the increased relative risk for oral/pharyngeal cancer in alcohol and tobacco users, it would seem prudent for the clinician to counsel patients about the need to decrease the frequency of smoking and drinking or, better yet, to quit smoking and drinking to excess.

Viruses

Several different viruses have been implicated in the development of human cancers with the differing viral genomes frequently found within cancers cells. By effecting oncogenes and other host cells' processes regulating cellular control, some viruses can effect cell proliferation, capabilities for invasion of surrounding structures, and apoptosis. The human immunodeficiency virus (HIV) is related to a number of different malignancy, some of which are defined as acquired immunodeficiency syndrome (AIDS)-defining malignancies. Some of the AIDS-defining or AIDS-related malignancies are found in the mouth and oropharynx. Other viruses, particularly the herpes viruses and human papilloma viruses (HPV), have been shown to cause cancers in several different organ systems. Although great progress has been seen over the last few decades, the complexity of the viral role in carcinogenesis is not understood completely. However, viruses do act, at least as cofactors, in several different malignancies. Hepatitis B and C have long been shown to have a direct correlation with hepatocellular carcinoma, especially when associated with chronic alcohol abuse. Human T-cell lymphotrophic virus has been shown to be etiologically associated with adult T-cell leukemia/lymphoma.

The herpes viruses have also been shown to have an association with cancer. Epstein-Barr virus (HHV-4, EBV) is a common virus that has been known to cause infectious mononucleosis and hairy leukoplakia. EBV also has been associated with Burkitt's lymphoma, certain Hodgkin's and non-Hodgkin's lymphomas, nasopharyngeal carcinoma, lymphomagenesis in immunocompromised patients, and posttransplantation lymphoproliferative disease [60–63]. Two Japanese studies have shown that EBV may be related to other oral cancers, including squamous cell carcinoma [64,65].

The herpes virus HHV-8 (KSHV) has been shown to cause tumors of the oral cavity. Kaposi's sarcoma (KS) is a predominantly vascular neoplasm, although there is often concomitant lymphatic proliferation. KS often begins as a purple macule that can progress to a plaque-like form [Fig. 4]. The flat forms of KS often progresses to a nodule and can progress to masses greater than 2 cm in diameter (tumor). Before the AIDS epidemic, Kaposi's sarcoma (KS) was a rare tumor most often found on the lower extremities of older men of Italian or eastern European decent. KS also is seen in gay men not infected with HIV (thought to be caused by as yet unidentified cofactors related to lifestyle), young black African men, prepubescent children, kidney transplant patients, and patients receiving immunosuppressive medications. The epidemic form of KS is the HIV-associated malignancy most often seen in the mouth. KS has been treated several different ways, including surgery, radiation therapy, and direct injection of cytotoxic drugs. Many KS lesions have been known to reduce in size when the patient is treated with highly active antiretroviral therapy (HAART).

Through its effect on immunosurveillence and actions as a cofactor with other viruses (including EBV and CMV) in development of oral/pharyngeal malignancies, HIV also has been associated with other "opportunistic" cancers. AIDS patients are at higher risk for developing non-Hodgkin's lymphomas [Fig. 5], conjunctival epithelial malignancies, cancers of the lip, testicular cancers (seminomas and nonseminomas), anal/rectal cancers, and lung and skin cancers. Oral/pharyngeal and tonsilar squamous cell

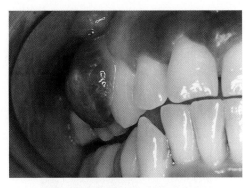

Fig. 4. Kaposi's sarcoma (35-year-old Caucasian male with AIDS diagnosis).

carcinomas [Fig. 6] also have been reported to occur more frequently in patients who have received an AIDS diagnosis [66,67].

More than 100 different HPVs are identified presently. HPV can be transmitted through sexual contact, including oral sex. Infection with HPV most often causes benign epithelial lesions (ie, genital warts, other papillomas). Notwithstanding the fact that most HPV-induced cellular changes are benign in their action, there are more than 10 HPVs which have been shown to cause cancers in a number of different mucosal surfaces. HPV-16, 18, 31, 33 and 35 have been shown to cause cancers of the uterine cervix, vulva, vagina, anus, and penis.

Infection with HPV also has been associated with oral squamous cell carcinoma. Although the relationship between oral squamous cell carcinoma and infection with HPV is unclear, HPV has been detected with increased frequency in oral dysplastic and carcinomatous epithelium when compared with normal epithelium [68,69].

Present data indicate that HPV plays at least a cofactor in oral squamous cell carcinoma development [70,71].

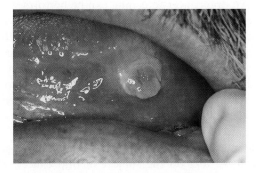

Fig. 5. Lymphoma (left lateral tongue, 47-year-old Caucasian male with AIDS diagnosis).

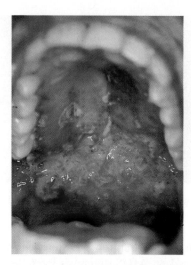

Fig. 6. Wide-spread squamous cell carcinoma involving entire soft palate (29-year-old African American male with AIDS diagnosis). This patient had concomitant squamous cell carcinoma of the rectum.

Vaccines have shown promise against certain types of HPV. A vaccine has recently been developed that can create host immunity for HPV16 and HPV18 and genital warts. Perhaps these vaccines also can be used in the future to reduce the incidence of HPV-associated oral malignancies.

Summary

Understanding the epidemiologic picture and the risk factors for oral cancer can help identify and treat patients at risk for oral cancers. Early diagnosis of an oral cancer continues to be important to achieving a favorable prognosis. Absent a diagnosis of oral/pharyngeal cancer, there clearly cannot be an effective treatment plan. Discovering a potentially malignant or malignant lesion and through biopsy reaching a diagnosis for the lesion begins by performing an examination with the purpose of detecting oral/pharyngeal lesions. An oral cancer screening can be performed in less than five minutes without any expensive diagnostic aids. Despite the ease with which this exam can be performed and the noninvasive nature of the examination, most patients report that they have never had an oral cancer examination. Late stage diagnosis continues to be a common situation resulting in high rates of morbidity and mortality. Without early recognition it seems that the trend of late stage diagnosis will continue. Physicians, dentists, and other health care providers should be performing the oral cancer screening examination on a routine basis for all of their patients.

Note: For the interested clinician, the author highly recommends an excellent comprehensive text on the subject of oral cancer. Sol Silverman's (with multiple contributors) The American Cancer Society's Atlas of

Clinical Oncology Oral Cancer: Fifth Edition by BC Decker Publishers is an excellent overview of oral cancer covering in greater detail many of the subjects that could not be covered in this brief article. Additionally, there are excellent color photographs of the common presentations of oral malignancies that can be helpful in assessing oral/pharyngeal lesions.

References

[1] Ries LAG, Eisner MP, Kosary CL, et al. Edwards Bk, editor. SEER cancer statistics review. Bethesda (MD): National Cancer Institute; 1975–2002.

[2] Shiboski CH, Shiboski SC, Silverman S. Trends in oral cancer rates in the United States, 1973–1996. Com Dent Oral Epidem 2000;28(4):249–56.

[3] Silverman S. Demographics and occurrence of oral and pharyngeal cancers. The outcomes, the trends, the challenge. J Am Dent Assoc 2001;132(Suppl):7S–11S.

[4] Silverman S. American cancer society atlas of clinical oncology. Oral Cancer. 5th edition. Hamilton, Ontario, Canada: BC Decker; 2003. p. 1–2.

[5] Moore SR, Johnson NW, Pierce AM, et al. The epidemiology of mouth cancer: a review of global incidence. Oral Dis 2000;6(2):65–74.

[6] Franceschi S, Bidoli E, Herrero R, et al. Comparison of cancers of the oral cavity and pharynx worldwide: etiological clues. Oral Oncol 2000;36(1):106–15.

[7] Mignogna MD, Felele S, Russo LL. The World Cancer Report and the burden of oral cancer. Eur J Cancer Prev 2004;13(2):139–42.

[8] Howell RE, Wright BA, Dewar R. Trends in the incidence of oral cancer in Nova Scotia from 1983 to 1997. Oral Surg Oral Med Oral Pathol Oral Radiol Endod 2003;95(2):205–12.

[9] Wunsch-Filho V. The epidemiology of oral and pharynx cancer in Brazil. Oral Oncol 2002; 38(8):737–46.

[10] Bosetti C, Franceschi S, Negri E, et al. Changing socioeconomic correlates for cancers of the upper digestive tract. Ann Oncol 2001;12(3):327–30.

[11] Mignogna MD, Fedele S, Russo LL. The World Cancer Report and the burden of oral cancer. Eur J Cancer Prev 2004;13(2):139–42.

[12] Zavras AI, Laskaris C, Kitta C, et al. Leukoplakia and intraoral malignancies. Female cases increase in Greece. J Eur Acad Dermatol Venereol 2003;17(1):25–7.

[13] O'Sullivan EM. Oral and pharyngeal cancer in Ireland. Ir Med J 2005;98(4):102–5.

[14] Llewellyn CD, Johnson NW, Warnakulasuriya KA. Risk factors for oral cancer in newly diagnosed patients aged 45 years and younger: a case-control study in Southern England. J Oral Pathol Med 2004;33(9):525–32.

[15] Tarvainen L, Suuronen R, Linqvist C, et al. Is the incidence of oral and pharyngeal cancer increasing in Finland? An epidemiological study of 17,383 cases in 1953–1999. Oral Dis 2004; 10(3):167–72.

[16] Iamaroon A, Pattanaporn K, Pongsiriwet S, et al. Analysis of 587 cases of oral squamous cell carcinoma in northern Thailand with a focus on young people. Int J Oral Maxillofac Surg 2004;33(1):84–8.

[17] Nevill BW, Damm DD, Allen CM, et al. Oral and maxillofacial pathology. Philadelphia: WB Saunders; 2002. p. 356.

[18] Iype EM, Pandey M, Mathew A, et al. Oral cancer in patients under the age of 35 years. J Postgrad Med 2002;47(3):171–6.

[19] Myers JN, Elkins T, Roberts D, et al. Squamous cell carcinoma of the tongue in young adults: increasing incidence and factors that predict treatment outcomes. Arch Otolaryngol Head Neck Surg 2000;122:44–51.

[20] Pitman KT, Johnson JT, Wagner RL, et al. Cancer of the tongue in patients less than forty. Head Neck 2000;22:297–302.

[21] Schantz SP, Yu GP. Head and neck cancer incidence trends in young Americans, 1973–1997, with special emphasis for tongue cancer. Arch Otolaryngol Head Neck Surg 2002;128(3): 268–74.

[22] Sugerman PB, Savage NW. Oral cancer in Australia. Aust Dent J 2002;47(1):45–56.

[23] de Boer MF, Sanderson RJ, Damhuis RA, et al. The effects of alcohol and smoking upon the age, anatomic sites and stage in the development of cancer of the oral cavity and oropharynx in females in the south west Netherlands. Eur Arch Otorhinolaryngol Suppl 1997;54(4): 177–9.

[24] Day GL, Blot WJ. Second primary tumors in patients with oral cancer. Cancer 1992;70(1): 14–9.

[25] Shibuya H, Wakita T, Nakagawa T, et al. The relation between an esophageal cancer and associated cancers in adjacent organs. Cancer 1995;76(1):101–5.

[26] Kramer FJ, Janssen M, Eckardt A. Second primary tumors in oropharyngeal squamous cell carcinoma. Clin Oral Investig 2004;8(2):56–62.

[27] Tomek MS, McGuirt WF. Second head and neck cancers and tobacco usage. Am J Otolaryngol 2003;24(1):24–7.

[28] Centers for Disease Control and Prevention. Tobacco use among middle and high school students—United States, 2002. MMWR 2003;52:1096–8.

[29] Marx RE, Stern D. Oral and maxillofacial pathology: a rationale for diagnosis and treatment. Chicago: Quintessence Publishing; 2003. p. 287.

[30] Rahman M, Sakamoto J, Fukui T. Bidi smoking and oral cancer: a meta-analysis. Int J Cancer 2003;106(4):600–4.

[31] Yaday JS, Thakus S. Cytogenetic damage in bidi smokers. Nicotine Tob Res 2000;2(1): 97–103.

[32] Wu W, Song S, Ashley DL, et al. Assessment of tobacco-specific nitrosamines in the tobacco and mainstream smoke of Bidi cigarettes. Carcinogenesis 2004;25(2):283–7.

[33] Malson JL, Lee EM, Murty R, et al. Clove cigarette smoking: biochemical, physiological and subjective effects. Pharmacol Biochem Behav 2003;74(3):739–45.

[34] Yen KL, Hechavarria E, Bostwick SB. Bidi cigarettes: an emerging thread to adolescent health. Arch Pediatr Adolesc Med 2000;154(12):1187–9.

[35] Allen JA, Vallone D, Haviland ML, et al. Tobacco use among middle and high school students—United States, 2002. MMWR 2003;52(45):1096–8.

[36] Celebucki C, Turner-Bowker DM, Connolly G, et al. Bidi use among urban youth—Massachusetts, March–April 1999. MMWR 1999;48(36):796–9.

[37] Bidis and Kreteks—Fact sheet July 2004. Tobacco Information and Prevention Source. Centers for Disease Control. Available at: http://www.cdc.gov/tobacco/factsheets/ bidisandkreteks.htm.

[38] Mangunnegro H, Sutoyo DK. Environmental and occupational lung diseases in Indonesia. Respirology 1996;1:85–93.

[39] Council on Scientific Affairs. Evaluation of the health hazard of clove cigarettes. JAMA 1988;260(24):3641–4.

[40] Franceschi S, Barra S, La Vecchia C, et al. Risk factors for cancer of the tongue and the mouth. A case-control study from northern Italy. Cancer 1992;70(9):2227–33.

[41] Marx RE, Stern D. Oral and maxillofacial pathology: a rationale for diagnosis and treatment. Chicago: Quintessence Publishing; 2003. p. 286.

[42] Bouquot JE, Meckstroth RL. Oral cancer in a tobacco-chewing US population—no apparent increased incidence or mortality. Oral Surg Oral Med Oral Pathol Oral Radiol Endod 1998;86(6):697–706.

[43] Foulds J, Ramstrom L, Burke M, et al. Effect of smokeless tobacco (snus) on smoking and public health in Sweden. Tob Control 2003;12(4):349–59.

[44] Accortt NA, Waterbor JW, Beall C, et al. Chronic disease mortality in a cohort of smokeless tobacco users. Am J Epidemiol 2002;156(8):730–7.

[45] Win DM, Blot WJ, Shy CM, et al. Snuff dipping and oral cancer among women in the southern United States. N Engl J Med 1981;304(13):745–9.
[46] Public Health Service. The health consequences of using smokeless tobacco: a report of the advisory committee of the Surgeon General. Bethesda (MD): US Department of Health and Human Services, Public Health Service; 1986. NIH publication no. 86–2874.
[47] International agency for research on cancer. Tobacco habits other than smoking; betel-quid and areca-nut chewing; and some related nitrosamines. Lyon, France: World Health Organization, International Agency for Research on Cancer; 1985. IARC monographs on the evaluation of the carcinogenic risk of chemicals to humans. Vol. 37.
[48] Hoffmann D, Djordjevic MV. Chemical composition and carcinogenicity of smokeless tobacco. Adv Dent Res 1997;11(3):322–9.
[49] Winn DM. Epidemiology of cancer and other systemic effects associated with the use of smokeless tobacco. Adv Dent Res 1997;111(3):313–21.
[50] Mashberg A, Garfinkle L, Harris S. Alcohol as a primary risk factor in oral squamous cell carcinoma. CA Cancer J Clin 1981;31:146–55.
[51] Franceshi S, Barra S, La Vecchia C, et al. Risk factors for cancer of the tongue and mouth. A case-control study from northern Italy. Cancer 1992;70(9):2227–33.
[52] Keller AZ. Alcohol, tobacco and age factors in the relative frequency of cancer among males with and without liver cirrhosis. Am J Epidemiol 1977;106:194–202.
[53] Blot WJ, McLaughlin JK, Winn DM, et al. Smoking and drinking in relation to oral and pharyngeal cancer. Cancer Res 1988;48(11):3282–7.
[54] Oliver AJ, Helfrick JF, Gard D. Primary oral squamous cell carcinoma: a review of 92 cases. J Oral Maxillofac Surg 1996;54(8):949–54.
[55] Macek MD, Reid BC, Yellowitz JA. Oral cancer examinations among adults at high risk: findings from the 1998 National Health Interview Survey. J Public Health Dent 2003;63(2):119–25.
[56] Shiu MN, Chen TH. Impact of betel quid, tobacco and alcohol on three-stage disease natural history or oral leukoplakia and cancer: implication for prevention of oral cancer. Eur J Cancer Prev 2004;13(1):39–45.
[57] Schildt EB, Eriksson M, Hardell L, et al. Oral snuff, smoking habits and alcohol consumption in relation to oral cancer in a Swedish case-control study. Int J Cancer 1998;77(3):341–6.
[58] Franceschi S, Bidoli E, Herrero R, et al. Comparison of cancers of the oral cavity and pharynx worldwide: etiological clues. Oral Oncol 2000;36(1):106–15.
[59] Franceshi S, Levi F, Dal Maso L, et al. Cessation of alcohol drinking and risk for cancer of the oral cavity and pharynx. Int J Cancer 2000;85(6):787–90.
[60] Cesarman E. Epstein-Barr virus (EBV) and lymphomagenesis. Front Biosci 2002;7:58–65.
[61] Cornelissen JJ. Molecular monitoring of EBV-positive lymphoma. Blood 2004;104(1):9.
[62] Au WY, Pang A, Choy C, et al. Quantification of circulating Epstein-Barr virus (EBV) DNA in the diagnosis and monitoring of natural killer cell and EBV-positive lymphomas in immunocompetent patients. Blood 2004;104:243–9.
[63] Thorley-Lawson DA, Gross A. Persistence of the Epstein-Barr virus and the origins of associated lymphomas. N Engl J Med 2004;350:1328–37.
[64] Shimkage M, Horii K, Tempaku A, et al. Association of Epstein-Barr virus with oral cancers. Hum Pathol 2002;33(6):608–14.
[65] Kobayashi I, Kaori S, Saito I, et al. Prevalence of Epstein-Barr virus in oral squamous cell carcinoma. J Pathol 1999;189(1):34–9.
[66] Flaitz CM, Nichols CM, Adler-Storthz K, et al. Intraoral squamous cell carcinoma in human immunodeficiency virus infection. Oral Surg Oral Med Oral Pathol Oral Radiol Endod 1995;80(1):55–62.
[67] Frisch M, Biggar RJ, Goedert JJ. Human papillomavirus-associated cancers in patient with human immunodeficiency virus infection and acquired immunodeficiency syndrome. J Natl Cancer Inst 2000;92(18):1500–10.

[68] Miller CS, Johnstone BM. Human papillomavirus as a risk factor for oral squamous cell carcinoma: a meta-analysis, 1982–1997. Oral Surg Oral Med Oral Pathol Oral Radiol Endod 2002;93(2):622–35.

[69] Kreimer AR, Clifford GM, Snijders PJ, et al. HPV16 semiquantitative viral load and serologic biomarkers in oral and oropharyngeal squamous cell carcinoma. Int J Cancer 2005; 115(2):329–32.

[70] Woods KV, Shillitoe EJ, Spitz MR, et al. Analysis of human papillomavirus DNA in oral squamous cell carcinoma. J Oral Pathol Med 1993;22(3):101–8.

[71] Herrero R, Castellsaque X, Pawlita M, et al. Human papillomavirus and oral cancer: the International Agency for Research on Cancer multicenter study. J Natl Cancer Inst 2003; 95(23):1772–83.

ELSEVIER
SAUNDERS

Otolaryngol Clin N Am
39 (2006) 295–306

OTOLARYNGOLOGIC
CLINICS
OF NORTH AMERICA

Early Diagnosis of Oral Cavity Cancers

Prairie Neeley Robinson, MD[a,*],
Alan R. Mickelson, PhD[b]

[a]*Department of Otolaryngology, University of Colorado Health Sciences Center,
4200 East 9th Avenue, B205, Denver, CO 80262, USA*
[b]*Department of Electrical and Computer Engineering, University of Colorado at Boulder,
Boulder, Colorado 80309-0425, USA*

Early diagnosis of carcinoma of the oral cavity is difficult to achieve. Between 1983 and 1990, 53% percent of patients with cancer of the oral cavity and pharynx demonstrated regional or distant metastasis at the time of diagnosis [1]. The 5-year survival rate is approximately 50% and has not improved in the last two decades. When lesions become symptomatic, patients complain of pain, bleeding, ulceration, a mass, dysphagia, or odynophagia; however, before the patient becomes symptomatic, the lesion is often growing and metastasizing.

Early diagnosis is rewarded with less morbidity and mortality. Physicians need to focus on screening patients considered to be at high risk and to act proactively to prevent morbidity and mortality from the disease process. Physicians should not wait for lesions to become symptomatic. There is a correlation between early diagnosis and an improved survival rate.

Regular screening is currently performed by dentists. Regular dental examinations have been included in the screening recommendations by the American Cancer Society; however, use of dental care by high-risk individuals is limited. One study indicated that patients were three times more likely to obtain care from a primary care physician than from a dentist before diagnosis [2].

Early detection

Physical examination

The high-risk sites of oral cavity carcinoma are the floor of the mouth, the ventrolateral tongue, the lingual aspect of the retromolar trigone, the

---

* Corresponding author. Otolaryngology, University of Colorado Health Science Center, 4200 East 9th Avenue, B205, Denver, CO 80262.

E-mail address: prairie.robinson@uchsc.edu (P.N. Robinson).

0030-6665/06/$ - see front matter © 2006 Elsevier Inc. All rights reserved.
doi:10.1016/j.otc.2005.12.001
oto.theclinics.com

palate, and the anterior tonsillar pillar. These areas are all easily visible on physical examination; therefore, early detection should initially focus on visual inspection of the oral cavity (Fig. 1). Otolaryngologists can examine the oral cavity as part of a routine head and neck examination in the office setting using a head mirror or light source and a laryngeal mirror to visualize areas that cannot be seen directly.

To evaluate the anterior oral cavity, the patient should open the mouth and raise the tip of the tongue, which should extend upward contacting the hard palate. To evaluate the posterior floor of mouth, the retromolar trigone, and the posterior ventrolateral tongue, the examiner should grasp the anterior one third of the tongue and pull anteriorly with a gauze sponge. A mirror can be used to visualize the lingual aspect of the retromolar trigone. The examination should also include palpation of mucosal surfaces and the neck for adenopathy.

The most common presentation of early squamous cell carcinoma is erythroplasia. Erythroplasia can appear as an innocuous lesion that is asymptomatic. The lesion is red in color, inflammatory, and atrophic. Erythroplasia is a common presentation of oral cavity cancers, especially in patients who smoke and drink.

In a study of 236 patients with asymptomatic oral carcinomas, 64% of the lesions were red, 12% were predominantly white, and 23% were equally white and red. The whitish color comes from keratin within the lesion. The mucosa can be heaped up but is not usually ulcerated. Asymptomatic lesions are usually less than 2 cm in diameter [3,4]. Some benign lesions are caused by an acute event or local factors. Nonneoplastic lesions usually subside within 14 days of the inciting event or the elimination of local factors.

A biopsy sample should be obtained from suspicious lesions. There is a higher diagnosis rate if the biopsy sample is obtained from the reddish part of the lesion versus the whitish, keratin-containing areas.

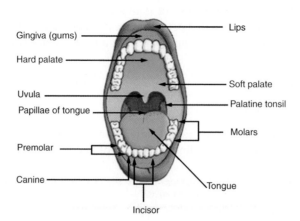

Fig. 1. Schematic anatomy of the oral cavity.

Leukoplakia is a whitish mucosal lesion that does not rub off and is not associated with any disease process. It is rarely precancerous. Only about 6% of early invasive carcinomas or carcinomas in situ have been shown to be purely white lesions [3,4]. Most carcinomas have a reddish component, which is an inflammatory response to the malignancy.

Lesions that are diagnosed later are usually painful to the patient, and the patient will complain of bleeding, pain, a mass, ulceration, dysphagia, or odynophagia. Larger later stage lesions are easily visible, and a biopsy sample should be obtained. Patients may also present with a neck mass, which is a regional metastasis from the oral cavity.

Vital staining

Physicians or dentists can employ other methods besides visual inspection on physical examination if they are suspicious of an area in the oral cavity or if a patient is considered high risk. Toluidine blue clinically stains malignant cells but not normal mucosa. There are two proposed mechanisms of toluidine blue staining. It is thought the dye is taken up by the nuclei of malignant cells manifesting increased DNA synthesis. Another hypothesis is that the dye can penetrate through randomly arranged tumor cells. Patients can rinse their mouths completely with the dye, and the physician can then inspect the areas for blue staining. Malignant lesions stain dark blue. Dysplastic lesions stain different shades of blue depending on the degree of dysplasia. Blue staining in a patient indicates the need for a biopsy.

Normal mucosa does not absorb toluidine blue stain. Occasionally, a small amount of dye may be retained in normal mucosa. This dye can be wiped away with acetic acid. Surfaces that are rough or keratinous will also hold stain (eg, the dorsum of the tongue, gingival crevices). Nonmalignant areas of inflammation occasionally stain with toluidine blue; therefore, all positive lesions should be restained in 14 days to decrease the false-positive rate.

Toluidine blue can also be used to screen patients who have had a carcinoma of the upper aerodigestive tract. These patients are known to be at high risk for a recurrence; therefore, clinicians may add toluidine rinses to their visual examination. Adding such rinses increases the sensitivity of detecting a lesion from 26.6% by visual inspection alone to 96.7% with toluidine blue staining [5].

Spectral analysis of oral tissue

A different technique that is showing promise for the early detection of oral carcinoma is spectral analysis [6–8], which is still in the early stages of clinical testing. Unlike visual methods, spectral techniques promise detection of precancerous conditions well before there is any visually detectable morphologic change such as the formation of a lesion.

There are numerous variations of the spectral detection technique. The basic idea is that a source of electromagnetic radiation is used to illuminate an area of oral tissue that is observed by a detection system that records the (wavelength) spectrum of the radiation that leaves the area of illumination during and immediately after the illumination period. The application of spectral detection to biosensing is not a new development. Previous applications have included an early multichannel blood oximeter [9], a later more portable oximeter [10], and an early portable diffuse reflectometer [11]. Advances in light emission and detection technology and new understanding of the mechanisms of molecular biology are serving as drivers for the application of spectral detection techniques in chemistry and biology in general and to early detection of oral cancer in particular.

One of the parameters that define the specific implementation of the spectral detection method is the center wavelength of the source or sources. The radiation may be ultraviolet (UV) [12], visible (VIS) [13], near infrared (NIR) [14], or, more recently, far infrared (FIR) or even TeraHertz (THz). The modulation applied to the source is another of the many variable parameters. The illumination in all cases is turned on and off, but the illumination period may vary from tiny fractions of a trillionth of a second (femtosecond pulse illumination) [15] to a quasi-steady illumination with a duration of possibly seconds [16]. There may be a single source [17] or as many as tens of sources, and these sources may illuminate the sample simultaneously or one at a time [18]. The detection system is also multivariate and may consist of a single detector or multiple detectors. The spectral recording system at the detector output may be a spectrometer or spectrum analyzer or may consist of filters and photon counters. The spectral region scanned may include the incident wavelength and wavelengths around the excitation wavelength [19] or may be tuned for the second of higher harmonics of the radiation [20,21]. Depending on the source modulation, the detection may be synchronous heterodyne, synchronous homodyne, or may use the simplest form of direct detection.

A multitude of systems have been devised and demonstrated. For the purposes of this review, the discussion is limited to some common features of the collected radiation, how they relate to the state of the tissue sampled, and why this technique might offer hope for detecting a premalignant condition long before it has the possibility of tumor metastasis or even before generating an affected field. The authors' group has been performing experimental and theoretical investigations of this technique as well as publishing studies. The apparatus used shares characteristics with a device described by Hart and JiJi [16] that is used primarily for sensing trace chemicals in water by using excitations from the near ultraviolet (NUV) through the VIS. Although we do not discuss our experimental or theoretical results herein, the research findings may affect the choice of materials to present and speculations about the cause and effects as well as predictions for the future.

Properties of tissue that allow for spectral diagnosis

The principle behind the operation of in vivo spectral analysis of tissue is that tissue is an inhomogeneous medium whose average index of refraction is not greatly different from any number of semitransparent materials. One can couple light into tissue because the material is somewhat index matched to the air, better than usual window glass at any rate, despite the fact that tissue is generally more absorptive than window glass. One can see the light that exits tissue because the inhomogeneity of the tissue causes it to scatter electromagnetic radiation of interesting wavelengths more strongly than it absorbs that radiation. The relevant parameter values of various tissue types are discussed in more detail in the article by Mourant and coworkers [22]. Tissue is to a great degree composed of water, in fact, 70% by weight. Water has an optical index of refraction near 1.33. There may be voids in tissue, but they are small. The fluid that makes up tissue is generally filled with sugars, fatty acids, amino acids, and nucleic acids, and the polymers (eg, polysaccharides, lipids, proteins, DNA, RNA) formed of these materials. The average index is higher than that of water and varies among cellular fluid (cytosol), structures within the cell (eg, mitochondria, endoplasmic reticula, Golgi apparati, lysosomes), nuclear cell material, and connective tissue. The index contrasts are the cause of the scattering that allows one to "see" into tissue.

After radiation incident on tissue has passed into tissue and begins to propagate, three processes can occur: scattering, absorption, and re-emission after absorption. The light can be scattered; the light can be absorbed; and, after absorption, there is some probability that the light can be re-emitted. The radiation is received by a detector after having been scattered from the tissue some number of times, or is scattered by the tissue some number of times before being absorbed, re-emitted, and then perhaps scattered multiple times again before being collected by the detector. The scattering, absorption, and re-emission (fluorescence) are all wavelength-dependent processes. Knowledge of the spectrum of the incident light and the received light can yield a wealth of data about the scattering parameters of the tissue, the absorption properties of the tissue, and the re-emission (often called fluorescent or luminescent) properties of the tissue. Spectral features of the fluorescence, absorption, and scattering are the parameters used to determine information about the state of the tissue.

Scattering

The lower row of pictures in Fig. 2 shows the lateral surface of the oral mucosa from the epical surface down to the basement basal membrane and some of the lateral surface of that submucosal layer for a series of cases of hyperplasia, dysplasia, and cancer. This section considers the general properties of the mucosa and its underlying layers for nominally healthy tissue. A subsequent section discusses how these properties are affected by the occurrence of neoplasia. Light incident from above the lateral strata in Fig. 2 will first encounter the squamous epithelial layer followed by the basement membrane, the stromal layer supporting the basement membrane, and then, below that stromal layer (not pictured in Fig. 2), a layer that contains blood vessels and their supporting tissue. Blood hemoglobin is absorptive and the layer supporting the vessels highly scattering. Although the scattering and absorption coefficients of the tissue (on the order of several per millimeter) allow a significant fraction of the incident light to traverse the mucosa (roughly 100 μm in thickness) and the millimeter of submucosa, the light is returned only weakly from the deeper layer.

The mucosal layer consists of a squamous epithelial layer and its basement layer. The squamous layer consists primarily of squamous cells. Associated with healthy squamous cells is an intracellular and extracellular matrix made up of various proteins including keratin, actin, and collagen. The inside of a squamous cell (and other somatic cells) is filled with cytoplasm as well as a cell nucleus and numerous other structures such as mitochondria, Golgi apparati, endoplasmic reticula, lysosomes, and peroxisomes. There is also a certain amount of keratin-rich material that is generated during the cell's lifetime. This keratin-rich material becomes the dominant material remaining in the cell as the squamous epithelial cell approaches apoptosis. A squamous cell may be approximately 10 μm in radius, whereas the nucleus may be 3 μm and other inner cellular structures yet smaller but still on the order of a wavelength of visible light (approximately 0.5 μm) or larger. The cytoplasm, in general, will have a refractive index moderately larger than that of water. For a wavelength at which the optical index of water is 1.33, the cell (apart from the nucleus and subnuclear structures) will have an index on the order of 1.34 to 1.35. The nucleus and other structures may have significantly higher indices, on the order of 1.40 or higher. These indices of 1.40 or higher are also characteristic of biopolymers such as proteins and the hydrophobic lipid bilayers of cell membranes. The squamous layer looks to an incident wave as a weakly scattering medium. The structures are larger than an optical wavelength, but their optical sizes, that is, the index relative to the background index (index contrast is $1.40 - 1.35 = 0.05$) multiplied by the actual size (<5 μm), are less than the incident wavelength (varies from 0.3 μm in the NUV to 1 μm or more in the NIR). One would expect that the scattering from such a medium would be spatially redistributed according to the Heney-Greenstein function, and such behavior has been reported [22].

The submucosal layer consists of numerous cell types. The strength of the layer is due to the long collagen fibers that crisscross the latter parallel to the mucosal surface. Such a crisscrossed layer can be referred to as a lamina propria [23]. These collagen fibers are hollow and have an index contrast on the order of the nuclei from the cell. The outer diameter of these layered collagen fibers can be approximately several micrometers, but the fibers can be much longer than they are thick. They can scatter more strongly than cell nuclei owing to their length.

Absorption and fluorescence

Cells and their supporting media can give rise to absorption. Mitochondria may be small, but they are hosts to energy-pumping reactions. NADH is one of the molecules that take part in energy storage and production processes. NADH absorbs strongly in the NUV and re-emits in the blue-green portion of the spectrum. Collagen, which is actually a protein, also is an autofluorescent species that absorbs NUV and emits (as it must) lower energy photons in the blue or blue-green portion of the spectrum. There are numerous other absorbing and emitting species such as tryptophan, elastin, and various flavins. Tryptophan has lines (absorption and emission) that lie in the NUV. Flavins absorb in the green and emit in the green-red portion of the spectrum. Because hemoglobin has the strongest absorption in the green portion of the spectrum, a sample with a lot of blood may mask the presence of flavins. In the study by Chen and coworkers [15], time-resolved fluorescence at a wavelength of 633 nm (0.633 μm) was monitored and correlated with the observed histopathology of the monitored region. The specific source of the 633 nm radiation was not mentioned.

Induced changes in the spectral properties of mucosa

Fig. 2 illustrates the lateral surface of the oral mucosa from the epical surface down to the basement basal membrane for tissue that exhibits hyperplasia, various states of dysplasia, and squamous cell carcinoma. The appearance of the hyperplastic tissue is actually similar to that of normal healthy mucosa. Healthy epithelial mucosa of the mouth consists of squamous cells that are aligned parallel to the epical and basement surfaces, as

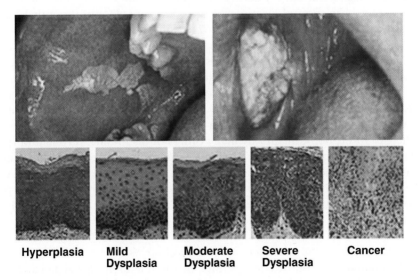

| Hyperplasia | Mild Dysplasia | Moderate Dysplasia | Severe Dysplasia | Cancer |

Fig. 2. Macroscopic and microscopic pictures of a series of cases of hyperplasia, dysplasia, and cancer of the oral mucosa.

seen in certain other mucosa such as that of the cervix or the outer skin layer. Order is imposed on the epithelial layer by the existence of intracellular and extracellular matrices consisting of an intricate and extensive system of protein structures made up of predominantly fine (nanometric) yet strong filaments. The components of the intracellular and extracellular matrices are not directly observable optically but have an effect on the optical properties of the boundaries between different index regions through changes in the boundary condition satisfied by the electric field component of the incident radiation field. At the lower boundary of healthy mucosa, there is a basal layer where the cells are oval or round rather than flattened. The epithelial stem cells that constantly replace upper epithelial cells that are shed into the oral cavity are located in this basal cell layer. It is speculated that the stem cells are located near cusps in the basement membrane. Lesions grow upward from the basement membrane. The fact that the basement membrane is not visible is one of the main reasons why it is so hard to detect cancers in their early stages. Once a lesion extends from the basement to the epical surface, the cancer has had a significant time to act.

Spectral properties of normal oral mucosa

For definiteness, let us consider the spectral properties of tissue in the NUV, VIS, and NIR regions of the "optical" spectrum. The preprocessing of multispectral techniques generally includes, first, the combination of the responses from the individual sources into an excitation emission matrix [13], and, second, a subsequent separation of the excitation emission matrix into individual fluorescence, absorbance, and scattering responses. The light returned from a normal epithelial layer will show fluorescent emission lines in the blue. The spectral locations of these lines are close to those that one might associate with collagen and NADH [6]. The scattering coefficient of the mucosa for the light is stronger in the blue and decreases monotonically to the red. This scattering coefficient is on the order of 2.5 mm in midrange. This effect is what would be expected to result from a random scattering medium where the optical sizes (index contrast multiplied by physical size) of particles are less than a wavelength. The variation of the scattering with wavelength is less than about an order of magnitude in the range of interest, whereas absorption can vary by many orders of magnitude. Strong absorption from a region where NADH should absorb may exceed the scattering value near the peak of its absorption. The NUV or blue excitations may be absorbed by NADH before reaching lower layers. There is also absorption from a spectral region where one would expect collagen to absorb, that is, in the NUV.

Spectral properties in cancerous and precancerous tissue

Examination of the row of pictures of the lateral epithelial mucosa in Fig. 2 indicates that the most noticeable morphologic change of the approach to cancer from a healthy state is the loss of structure of the mucosal layer. As the cells lose their squamous forms, they enlarge and become amorphous in shape. As shown in the report by Wang and coworkers [23], keratin can actually appear in intercellular pearls rather than in highly ordered lines between intracellular desmosomes. The morphologies of the layers as one observes a progression from normal epithelium toward a cancerous one increase in their configurational entropies.

Various investigators have concentrated attention on the autofluorescence spectrum and its changes when considering the spectral diagnosis of cancer. A common observation is that the shape of the blue fluorescence features changes [6–8]. Muller and coworkers [6] attribute this change to a decrease in the contribution of the collagen fluorescence and a small increase in the contribution of the NADH fluorescence. When noted, it has been reported that the scattering of the medium decreases along with an increase of absorption. The changes in fluorescence and absorption may proceed any morphologic changes. Although there may be other signals that one could also concentrate on [24], NADH and collagen seem to be the native fluorophores that exhibit the most easily observable changes.

The direction of spectral detection research

As pointed out by de Veld and coworkers [8], there is a need to improve on the specificity and sensitivity of spectral detection techniques. de Veld and colleagues believe that the white light sources they are using to generate spectral launches are not the proper approach, and, indeed, most groups involved in such research agree that laser [6,13,15] or light-emitting diode techniques [16] are more viable sources to employ to achieve the necessary specificities and sensitivities.

Other screening modalities

Another screening tool is a product called ViziLite [25]. ViziLite (Zila Pharmaceuticals, Phoenix, Arizona) is a screening tool targeted at dentists to assist in the identification of cancerous oral cavity tissue. It consists of an acetic acid wash and a single use "chemi-light stick" that generates a moderately short wavelength source for illumination of the oral cavity. ViziLite product literature claims up to 30% specificity. The hypothesis behind the ViziLite product is that the density of the nuclear content and mitochondrial matrix of abnormal cells is typically greater than that of normal cells. The increased molecular density may reveal the increased proliferative rate and metabolic activity of precancerous cells. ViziLite examination enhances the examiner's ability to see the difference in the nuclear to cytoplasmic ratio of dysplastic cells. After the patient rinses with a dilute acetic acid solution, the dense nucleus of abnormal squamous epithelium tissue will appear white when viewed under a diffuse low-energy wavelength light. Normal epithelium will absorb the light and appear dark. ViziLite can identify an abnormality, but a definitive diagnosis can only be made by biopsy [25]. One study in Malaysia compared toluidine blue rinses with ViziLite in high-risk patients and found a sensitivity of 100% and a specificity of 14.2% for ViziLite. In the same study, toluidine blue had a sensitivity of 70.3% and a specificity of 25%. ViziLite and toluidine blue were equal in terms of detecting cases of squamous cell carcinoma. ViziLite was better than toluidine blue rinses at picking up dysplastic lesions but also reacted to oral lichen planus, which increased the false-positive rate for ViziLite [25].

Physicians and dentists can use an oral brush to obtain cells from a suspicious area of the oral cavity to avoid the pain and discomfort of a tissue biopsy. A product called OralCDx Brush Biopsy (CDx Laboratories, Suffern, New York) includes an abrasive brush used to collect oral tissue. The thought behind this brush biopsy is to allow dentists or physicians to sample benign but questionable lesions in the office. The OralCDx Brush Biopsy is not used when a lesion is extremely suspicious or large. A formal biopsy is still indicated if there is clinical suspicion of a lesion regardless of the OralCDx result [26].

Controversy exists over the use of the OralCDx product because some studies have indicated a high false-positive and high false-negative rate. In a study of 298 cases, there were 4 false-negative results and 150 false-positive results [27]. The false-negative rate could delay a necessary scalpel biopsy. Nevertheless, other studies comparing the OralCDx product with histologic findings have found a sensitivity of 92.3% and a specificity of 94.3% in 103 patients [28] and a sensitivity of over 96% and a specificity of 90% in 945 patients. There are multiple examples in the literature of studies with essentially opposite findings; therefore, most articles suggest further investigation of the product.

Summary

Dentists, primary care physicians, and otolaryngologists should continue to perform complete oral cavity examinations and should be aware of high-risk populations for oral cavity carcinomas. Oral cavity carcinoma is the sixth most common cancer and is often detected in later stages. By using the modalities of physical examination, brush biopsies, vital staining, and spectral analysis, it is hoped that more cancers will be detected at an early stage, decreasing the morbidity and mortality of oral cavity tumors.

References

[1] Wingo PA, Tong T, Bolden S. Cancer statistics 1995. CA Cancer J Clin 1995;45:8–30.
[2] Prout MN, Herreen TC, Barber CE, et al. Use of health services before diagnosis of head and neck cancer among Boston residents. Am J Prev Med 1990;6:77–83.
[3] Mashberg A, Feldman LJ. Clinical criteria for identifying early oral and oropharyngeal carcinoma: erythroplasia revisited. Am J Surg 1988;152:351–3.

[4] Mashberg A, Merletti F, Boffetta P, et al. Appearance, site of occurrence and physical and clinical characteristics of oral carcinoma in Torino, Italy. Cancer 1989;63:2522–7.

[5] Epstein JB, Feldman R, Dolor RJ, et al. The utility of tolonium chloride rinse in the diagnosis of recurrent or second primary cancers in patients with prior upper aerodigestive tract cancer. Head Neck 2003;25(11):911–21.

[6] Muller MG, Valdez TA, Georgakoudi I, et al. Spectroscopic detection and evaluation of morphologic and biochemical changes in early oral carcinoma. Cancer 2003;97(7):1681–92.

[7] de Veld DCG, Skurchina M, Witjes MJH, et al. Clinical study for classification of benign, dysplastic and malignant oral lesions using autofluorescence spectroscopy. J Biomed Optics 2004;9(5):940–50.

[8] de Veld DCG, Skurchina M, Witjes MJH, et al. Autofluorescence and diffuse reflectance spectroscopy for oral oncology. Lasers Surg Med 2005;36(5):356–64.

[9] Mayevsky A, Chance B. Intracellular oxidation-reduction state measured in situ by a multi-channel fiberoptic fluorometer. Science 1982;217(4559):537–40.

[10] Feather JW, Ellis DJ, Leslie G. A portable reflectometer for the rapid quantification of cutaneous haemoglobin and melanin. Phys Med Biol 1988;33(6):711–22.

[11] Osawa M, Niwa S-I. A portable diffuse reflectance spectrophotometer for rapid and automatic measurement of tissue. Meas Sci Technol 1993;4:668–76.

[12] Sacks PG, Savage HE, Levine J, et al. Native cellular fluorescence identifies terminal squamous differentiation of normal oral epithelial cells in culture: a potential chemoprevention biomarker. Cancer Lett 1996;104:171–81.

[13] Zangaro RA, Silviera L Jr, Manoharan R, et al. Rapid multiexcitation fluorescence spectroscopy for in vivo tissue diagnostics. Appl Optics 1996;35:5211–9.

[14] Cooney KM, Gossage KW, McShane MJ, et al. Development of an optical system for the detection of oral cancer using near-infrared spectroscopy. In: Proceedings of the 26th Annual International Conference of the IEEE in Medicine and Biology Society; 1998;20:906–9.

[15] Chen H-S, Chiang C-P, You C, et al. Time-resolved autofluorescence spectroscopy for classifying normal and premalignant oral tissues. Lasers Surg Med 2005;37:37–45.

[16] Hart SJ, JiJi RD. Light emitting diode excitation of emission matrix fluorescence spectroscopy. Analyst 2002;127:1693–9.

[17] Nieman LT, Myakov A, Sokolov K. Fiberoptic probe for reflectance spectroscopy: oral mucosa studies. In: Proceedings of the Second Joint EMBS/BMES Conference. Houston (TX); 2002. p. 2267–68.

[18] Park SY, Collier T, Aaron J, et al. Multispectral digital microscope for in vivo monitoring of oral neoplasia in the hamster cheek pouch model of carcinogenesis. Optical Express 2005; 13(3):749–62.

[19] Motz JT, Hunter M, Galindo LH, et al. Optical fiber probe for biomedical Raman spectroscopy. Appl Optics 2004;43(3):542–54.

[20] Wilder-Smith P, Osann K, Hanna N, et al. In vivo multiphoton fluorescence imaging: a novel approach to oral malignancy. Lasers Surg Med 2004;35:96–103.

[21] Skala MC, Squrrell JM, Vrotsos KM, et al. Multiphoton microscopy of endogenous fluorescence differentiates between normal, precancerous, and cancerous squamous epithelial tissues. Cancer Res 2005;65(4):1180–6.

[22] Mourant JR, Freyer JP, Hielscher AH, et al. Mechanisms of light scattering from biological cells relevant to noninvasive optical tissue diagnostics. Appl Optics 1998;37(16):3586–93.

[23] Wang C-Y, Tsai T, Chen H-M, et al. PLS-ANN based classification model for oral submucosus and oral carcinogenesis. Lasers Surg Med 2003;32:318–26.

[24] Kornberg LJ, Villaret D, Popp M, et al. Gene expression profiling in squamous cell carcinoma of the oral cavity shows abnormalities in several signaling pathways. Laryngoscope 2005;115:690–8.

[25] Ram S, Siar CH. Chemiluminescence as a diagnostic aid in the detection of oral cancer and potentially malignant epithelial lesions. Int J Oral Maxillofac Surg 2005;34(5):521–7.

[26] Joseph BK. Oral cancer: prevention and detection. Med Princ Pract 2002;11(Suppl 1):32–5.
[27] Svirsky JA, Burns JC, Carpenter WM, et al. Comparison of computer-assisted brush biopsy results with follow-up scalpel biopsy and histology. Gen Dent 2002;50:500–6.
[28] Scribba JJ, US Collaborative OralCDx Study Group. Improving detection of precancerous and cancerous oral lesions: computer-assisted analysis of the oral brush biopsy. J Am Dent Assoc 1999;130:1445–57.

ELSEVIER
SAUNDERS

Otolaryngol Clin N Am
39 (2006) 307–317

OTOLARYNGOLOGIC
CLINICS
OF NORTH AMERICA

Imaging of Oral Cancer

Laura Lee Simon, MD[a], David Rubinstein, MD[b],*

[a]3236 Country Club Parkway, Castle Rock, CO 80104, USA
[b]Department of Radiology, Campus Box A034, University of Colorado Health Sciences
Center, 4200 East 9th Avenue, Denver, CO 80206, USA

The imaging of oral cancers involves the evaluation of the primary neoplasm as well as searching the neck for metastases to lymph nodes. In most hospitals, primary oral neoplasms, like other head and neck neoplasms, usually are evaluated by CT and MRI. The search for lymph node metastases also is usually performed with one of these modalities. Positron emission tomography (PET) is usually reserved for equivocal cases in institutions where it is available. It can be used to evaluate the primary neoplasm and to search for metastases. Some institutions also use ultrasound (US) to evaluate lymph nodes. Each of these modalities may play a role in the full evaluation of a patient who has an oral neoplasm. In addition, several new techniques that may aid in the diagnosis and staging of oral malignancies are being evaluated.

Evaluation of the primary tumor

The evaluation of the primary neoplasm mainly involves determining the extent of the tumor and the involvement of adjacent structures that may include the mandible or carotid artery. The primary tumor is detected by distortion of the normal anatomy or by having imaging characteristics different from the normal adjacent tissue. CT was the first modality to allow reliable differentiation of head and neck neoplasms from normal neck anatomy.

The original CT scanners were able to produce a single slice with each rotation of the x-ray tube around the patient, producing an axial section every few minutes. With the increasing speed of computers, the scanners were able to produce an axial section in just a few seconds. In the early 1990s helical scanners became available that further increased the speed of the scanners, and in the late 1990s multidetector or multislice scanners were developed

* Corresponding author.

0030-6665/06/$ - see front matter © 2005 Elsevier Inc. All rights reserved.
doi:10.1016/j.otc.2005.11.007

that allow the acquisition of a volume of data. Scanners with 64 rows of detectors are now available, and 16-slice scanners are fairly common.

Standard CT imaging of the oral cavity and oropharynx, like CT imaging of the rest of the face and neck, should use a section thickness of no more than 5 mm. With multidetector CT, slice thicknesses of 0.5 to 3 mm are easily possible. Although CT has primarily been used for axial imaging in the past, the thin sections possible with multidetector CT make reformatted images in any plane a real possibility (Fig. 1). Coronal and sagittal reformatted images are now commonly used to evaluate all areas of the face and neck. The use of thinner collimation and high-definition algorithms has decreased bony and other artifacts in the evaluation of the head and neck.

Unless there is a contraindication to the administration of iodinated contrast, the study should be performed during the infusion of intravenous contrast. The contrast may make the neoplasm enhance and become more

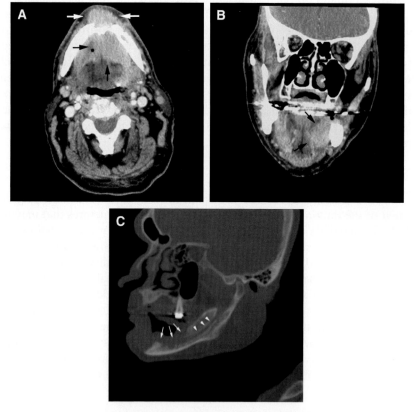

Fig. 1. (*A*) Axial and (*B*) coronal reformatted enhanced CT images demonstrate a fairly well-demarcated floor of mouth neoplasm (*arrows*) that is denser than adjacent tissue. (*C*) Oblique reformatted images through the mandible demonstrate bone destruction (*thin arrows*) and enlargement of the inferior alveolar canal or mandibular canal (*arrowheads*).

conspicuous against a background of less-enhancing structures. The contrast also makes it easier to distinguish between the brightly opacified vessels and lymph nodes.

Studies have shown that the use of CT is helpful for the evaluation of patients who have neoplasms of the head and neck [1,2]. CT is better able to determine the extent of neoplasm than clinical examination and can reveal lymph nodes that are not clinically apparent. For these reasons CT has become an essential part of the workup of patients who have oral neoplasms.

Neoplasms are detected on CT based on their density and morphology. Most oral neoplasms enhance and appear brighter than most other tissues except vessels (see Fig. 1). Some appear isodense to the surrounding tissue, and some, especially necrotic neoplasms (Fig. 2), are hypodense, at least in part. Isodense lesions can be detected if they distort the normal anatomy, indent the oropharyngeal airway, or obliterate expected fat planes. The sensitivity of CT for invasion of the mandible by an oral cavity neoplasm (see Fig. 1C) is 64%, but its specificity is 89% [3].

Imaging of the oral cavity may be difficult in patients who have dental amalgam or metallic dental devices. The amalgam or metal can cause artifact that obscures anatomy and pathology in the sections where the devices are included. The number of sections that are degraded by the artifact can be minimized by scanning parallel to the plane containing the metal. Scanning at multiple angles around the dental artifact can help in evaluating the more posteriorly located oropharynx. In this way, the entire oropharynx can usually be covered without artifact (Fig. 3). Anatomy and lesions located adjacent to the metallic material cannot be well evaluated, however.

MRI was developed after the CT scanner but more quickly became an established modality for the evaluation of neck and face neoplasms. MRI takes advantage of several physical characteristics of tissues to create images

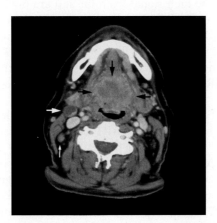

Fig. 2. Enhanced axial CT demonstrates a necrotic base of tongue neoplasm (*black arrows*) and a necrotic lymph node (*white arrow*) behind the right submandibular gland. An enlarged lymph node (*thin white arrow*) lies deep to the right sternocleidomastoid muscle.

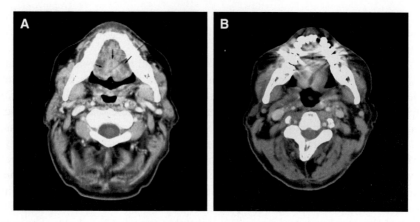

Fig. 3. (*A*) CT scan at one angle through the oral cavity demonstrates a tongue neoplasm (*arrows*). (*B*) A second section with a different scan angle has artifact from dental amalgam and does not show the neoplasm.

without the use of ionizing radiation. The density of protons, T1 relaxation time, and T2 relaxation times are the characteristics most frequently used for imaging. A routine MRI examination should include T2-weighted scans as well as T1-weighted scans performed both before and after the administration of contrast. Because MRI images can be generated in any plane, axial, coronal, and sagittal sequences should be performed.

Fat saturation may be used on postcontrast T1-weighted scans to make enhancing lesions more conspicuous, because without fat saturation both the enhancing lesions and fat are bright on T1-weighted scans. Fat saturation can also be helpful on T2-weighted scans, where neoplasms are usually hyperintense, as is fat. Inversion recovery scans can also demonstrate T2 weighting without the high signal from fat and are preferred by some radiologists over fat-saturated T2-weighted images [4,5]. As on CT, neoplasm can also be detected by distortion of the normal anatomy on MRI.

As with CT, the sections on MRI should not be thicker than 5 mm, and the field of view should be as small as possible but still include the entire neck and face. MRI sections as thin as 3 mm can be obtained on most scanners.

MRI also may be hindered by dental hardware. If dental hardware distorts the local magnetic fields, the MRI scans will be distorted. This distortion will affect the imaging in all planes. The amount of artifact seen on CT from dental devices may not correlate with the amount seen on MRI.

Because MRI uses strong magnetic and electromagnetic fields, special considerations must be made for patient safety. Medical devices or implants that can be moved in the magnetic field are a contraindication to MRI. These devices include ferromagnetic intracranial aneurysm clips and heart valves. Metallic foreign bodies can also be moved in the magnetic field and may cause harm. Patients are screened for metallic foreign bodies in the orbits where they can damage the globe and for shrapnel near vital organs, especially the brain and spinal cord. Cardiac pacemakers, neurostimulators, programmable ventricular shunts, infusion pumps, cochlear implants, and any mechanically, electrically, or magnetically controlled implant are also contraindications to MRI, although some devices may be reprogrammed after a MRI scan.

On MRI, neoplasms are usually brighter than the surrounding tissues on T2-weighted scans (Fig. 4A). The neoplasms may be isodense with other tissues on T1-weighted scans, but they usually enhance with contrast. As a result the neoplasms are brighter than the most surrounding tissue on enhanced scans (Fig. 4B).

Although both CT and MRI are widely used to evaluate oral neoplasms, MRI usually is better at demonstrating the extent of the primary [6,7]. MRI

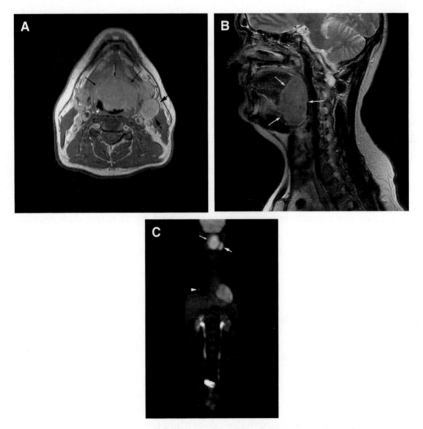

Fig. 4. (*A*) Enhanced axial T1-weighted and (*B*) sagittal T2-weighted MRI scans show a large tongue base neoplasm (*thin arrows*). The axial image (*A*) also demonstrates an enlarged metastatic lymph node (*arrow*). (*C*) A PET scan demonstrates the neoplasm (*thin arrow*) and the node (*arrow*). The PET scan also shows a small lung nodule (*arrowhead*) that could be benign, a second primary neoplasm, or a metastasis.

is more sensitive than CT for determining mandibular invasion (94% versus 64%) but is less specific (73% versus 89%) [3]. MRI is more expensive than CT, and the decision whether to evaluate neoplasms with CT, MRI, or both is usually made on a case-by-case basis.

PET is based on the metabolism of the neoplasm, whether primary, metastatic, or recurrent. PET scanning uses [18]fluorodeoxyglucose (FDG), a molecule that the body treats as glucose. The radiopharmaceutical is injected with the patient in a quiet room. The radiopharmaceutical is then distributed in the blood throughout the body and is taken up by the most metabolically active regions. The patient then is put in a coincidence scanner. A positron particle emitted from the radiopharmaceutical travels a short distance and then annihilates into two daughter photons that travel in opposite directions and strike the scanner at the same time (coincidence). A mathematical algorithm is used to determine the point of origin in the body. Although PET scanners are not universally available, they can be found at most major medical centers.

Neoplasms appear as regions of increased activity on PET scans (Fig. 4C), but not everything that has increased activity is neoplasm. Normal physiologic uptake of FDG must be differentiated from pathology. The salivary glands, nasal turbinates, lymphoid tissue, and any active muscles take up FDG to varying degrees and can be confused with neoplasm. Neoplasm adjacent to a normal structure with high FDG uptake can also be easily overlooked. Pathologic processes such as infection and inflammation have an appearance similar to neoplasm on PET scans.

PET does not seem to have a significant benefit in the preoperative evaluation of known primary neoplasms [6,8]. PET is, however, beneficial in the evaluating recurrent or residual neoplasm [9–11], especially when MRI or CT cannot distinguish between changes caused by therapy and neoplasm. Some believe the fusion of PET and CT will improve the performance of PET scans [12]. Combined PET/CT scanners are now becoming more available.

Evaluation of lymph nodes

As with the extent of the primary neoplasm, it has been shown that imaging is more sensitive than clinical examination for the detection of enlarged lymph nodes [13,14]. To detect metastases CT and MR usually use the imaging parameters used to evaluate the primary neoplasm. To search for metastases, the CT or MR examination is usually extended to cover the entire neck. PET scans usually cover the entire body, so the metastatic search is part of the examination for the primary neoplasm. In addition to those modalities, US also can be used to search for metastatic lymph nodes. Unfortunately, in most institutions none of the available imaging modalities are both highly specific and sensitive or, from the clinical viewpoint, have high positive and negative predictive values [15]. Each of the modalities has criteria for distinguishing benign from malignant adenopathy. CT and MRI use size as the primary criterion for determining if a lymph node contains a metastasis. Specificity may be improved, if imaging identifies necrosis or extracapsular spread. US uses size, internal architecture, and Doppler blood-flow pattern as the primary criteria, and PET scanning uses metabolic activity.

CT and MRI are the modalities most commonly used for the evaluation of lymph nodes. It is debatable whether CT or MRI is more accurate for determining if lymph nodes contain metastases, but neither is highly accurate [16,17]. Criteria for separating reactive from metastatic lymph nodes are the presence of necrosis, the presence of extracapsular spread, and size.

Necrosis is identified on CT as a region of decreased density within a lymph node on an enhanced study (see Fig. 2) [18,19]. Care must be taken not to mistake the normal fat in the hilum of the lymph node as a region of necrosis. On MRI necrosis appears as regions of poor or no enhancement within a lymph node [18] or of low signal [19] on T1-weighted scans and as regions of increased signal in a node on T2-weighted scans [18,19]. On any modality the lack of sharp borders around any node or invasion of surrounding tissue is a sign of extracapsular spread of neoplasm from the node [20]. Both necrosis and extracapsular spread are fairly specific for malignancy in the setting of a primary neoplasm, but neither is very sensitive for detecting malignant nodes.

The most commonly used size criterion for determining whether a lymph node is metastatic is 10 mm in the largest axial diameter, although other size criteria have been suggested [18,21]. Using a 10-mm maximal axial diameter and the identification of necrosis in nodes between the angle of the mandible and the cricoid cartilage, one study demonstrated that CT had a 90% sensitivity, a 38% specificity, an 84% negative predictive value, and a 50% positive predictive value for metastatic disease affecting a hemi-neck, whereas MRI scored 82%, 48%, 79%, and 52%, respectively, for the same tests. Dropping the size criterion to 5 mm, CT scored 98%, 13%, 90%, 44%, respectively, and MRI scored 92%, 20%, 77%, and 44%, respectively. The same study found that adding the information about necrosis did not significantly change the performance of CT or MRI when considering lymph nodes 10 mm or smaller [16].

Another study demonstrated that the ratio of the lengths of the maximal longitudinal and axial axes of a lymph node can provide an accurate method for detecting metastases. This study found a sensitivity and specificity of 97% for individual lymph nodes when a ratio of less than 2 was used to indicate a metastasis [22]. This criterion is not widely used, and the study has not been confirmed.

US is commonly used in Asia and Europe but not in the United States to evaluate for metastatic lymph nodes [23]. It has been suggested that US is better than CT for determining if a lymph node harbors a metastasis [24].

US can use several criteria for evaluating nodes. As on CT and MR, the size of the lymph node is an important criterion. The internal architecture and the pattern of blood flow in the node depicted with Doppler US are used in conjunction with the lymph node size. Presence of normal hilar echogenicity and a normal hilar pattern of flow suggest a benign lymph node. Metastatic lymph nodes can lose both the normal hilar architecture and blood flow [24]. One study suggests that the ratio of the largest-to-smallest diameters of the lymph node on US is a highly accurate way to detect metastatic lymph nodes [25]. US is highly user dependant, and the accuracy of the diagnosis of metastatic disease may be affected by the expertise of the person performing the examination.

PET uses metabolic activity to evaluate for metastatic lymph nodes. PET scans usually include the entire body and so may detect metastases distant from the neck [26,27] as well as second primary neoplasms (see Fig. 4C). It is unclear if PET is helpful for evaluation of metastatic nodes. Some studies have found PET helpful for staging head and neck cancers [8,28], whereas others find it of no benefit relative to CT, MRI, or US [15,29,30].

New techniques

In addition to the widely used imaging modalities, new techniques are being developed and evaluated. New MRI methods take advantage of increased speed of imaging techniques and physiologic differences between tissues.

Volumetric interpolated breath-hold examination (VIBE) is a gradient-echo MRI sequence first reported for abdominal imaging and since described as having utility in evaluating brain, abdominal, breast, and chest lesions. It allows short acquisition times (approximately one fifth to one tenth those of conventional spin-echo T1-weighted imaging) with resulting images that are comparable or superior to those obtained by conventional gradient-recalled echo sequences. In evaluations of the head and neck, VIBE-sequence MRI has been shown to be an acceptable alternative to postcontrast spin-echo T1-weighted imaging [31].

Functional imaging using dynamic contrast-enhanced MRI takes advantage of relative differences in the microcirculation of malignant and nonmalignant tissue to achieve increased contrast signal following administration of a contrast bolus. Theoretically, malignancy can be distinguished with greater confidence. The basic technique of dynamic contrast-enhanced MRI scans the area of interest multiple times. Imaging starts before contrast administration, continues through the contrast injection, and ends after the contrast bolus has been injected. This results in approximately three to four scanning sequences over an approximate 2- to 5-minute period.

Dynamic contrast-enhanced gradient-echo MR imaging has been demonstrated to be superior to conventional contrast-enhanced spin-echo imaging to delineate margins and extent of tumors visually [32]. Evaluation of lymph nodes with dynamic contrast-enhanced MRI and quantitative analysis found different enhancement patterns in metastatic neck nodes than in reactive nodes [33]. Despite the apparent successes of dynamic MRI, it is not widely used.

Diffusion-weighted imaging is an MRI sequence used to measure the ability of water molecules to diffuse in different tissues. It is most often used to detect acute infarcts in the brain, but it has been used to characterize lesions in the head and neck. One study found the amount of diffusion was different in different malignancies and was different in malignancies and in benign lesions [34]. Another study was able to discriminate between benign and malignant nodes [35]. Like dynamic MRI, the experimental success for diffusion-weighted imaging has not been followed by widespread clinical use.

Iron oxide enhanced MRI uses ultra-small superparamagnetic iron oxide (USPIO) particles that are administered intravenously and are concentrated in the reticuloendothelial system by functioning histiocytes in normal lymph nodes. Normal lymph nodes demonstrate reduced signal intensity on T2*-weighted gradient-echo and T2-weighted MR images. Lymph nodes that have been replaced or invaded by malignant cells do not take up the USPIO particles and consequently keep their precontrast signal intensity. These changes are progressive over 6 to 24 hours after administration of the contrast agent. It has been suggested that MRI with USPIO particles will increase the sensitivity and specificity for detecting metastatic nodes, but no definite improvement over CT and routine MR has been proven [36,37].

Although imaging of oral cavity cancer remains less than perfect, it is usually helpful in the initial evaluation and follow-up of patients who have these neoplasms.

References

[1] Larsson SG, Mancuso A, Hanafee W. Computed tomography of the tongue and floor of the mouth. Radiology 1982;143:493–500.
[2] Murakai AS, Mancuso AA, Harnsberger HR, et al. CT of the oropharynx, tongue base and floor of the mouth: normal anatomy and range of variations, and applications in staging carcinoma. Radiology 1983;148:725–31.
[3] van den Brekel MW, Runne RW, Smeele LE, et al. Assessment of tumor invasion of the mandible: the value of different imaging techniques. Eur Radiol 1998;8:1552–7.
[4] Nakatsu M, Hatabu H, Itoh H, et al. Comparison of short inversion time inversion recovery (STIR) and fat-saturated (chemsat) techniques for background fat intensity suppression for cervical and thoracic MR imaging. J Magn Reson Imaging 2000;11:56–60.
[5] Sadick M, Sadick H, Hormann K, et al. Diagnostic evaluation of magnetic resonance imaging with turbo inversion recovery sequence in head and neck tumors. Eur Arch Otorhinolaryngol 2005;262:634–9.
[6] Damman F, Horger M, Mueller-Berg M, et al. Rational diagnosis of squamous cell carcinoma of the head and neck region: comparative evaluation of CT, MR and 18FDG PET. AJR Am J Roentgenol 2005;184:1326–31.
[7] Leslie A, Fyfe E, Guest P, et al. Staging of squamous cell carcinoma in the oral cavity and oropharynx: a comparison of MRI and CT in T- and N-staging. J Comput Assist Tomogr 1999;23:43–9.

[8] Ng SH, Yen TC, Liao CT, et al. 18F-FDG PET and CT/MRI in oral cavity squamous cell carcinoma: a prospective study of 124 patients with histologic correlation. J Nucl Med 2005; 46:1136–43.

[9] Fischbein NJ, AAssar OS, Caputo GR, et al. Clinical utility of positron emission tomography with 18F-fluorodeoxyglucose in detecting residual/recurrent squamous cell carcinoma of the head and neck. AJNR Am J Neuroradiol 1998;19:1189–96.

[10] Kubota K, Yokoyama J, Yamaguchi K, et al. FDG-PET delayed imaging for the detection of head and neck cancer recurrence after radio-chemotherapy: comparison with MRI/CT. Eur J Nucl Med Mol Imaging 2004;31:590–5.

[11] Farber LA, Benard F, Machtay M, et al. Detection of recurrent head and neck squamous cell carcinomas after radiation therapy with 2–18F-fluoro-2-deoxy-D-glucose positron emission tomography. Laryngoscope 1999;109:970–5.

[12] Branstetter BF IV, Blodgett TM, Zimmer LA, et al. Head and neck malignancy: is PET/CT more accurate than PET or CT alone? Radiology 2005;235:580–6.

[13] Stevens MH, Harnsberger HR, Mancuso AA, et al. Computed tomography of cervical lymph nodes. Staging and management of head and neck cancer. Arch Otolaryngol 1985; 111:735–9.

[14] Haberal I, Celik H, Gocmen H, et al. Which is important in the evaluation of metastatic lymph nodes in head and neck cancer: palpation, ultrasonography or computed tomography? Otolaryngol Head Neck Surg 2004;130:197–201.

[15] Stuckensen T, Kovacs AF, Adams S, et al. Staging of the neck in patients with oral cavity squamous cell carcinomas: a prospective comparison of PET, ultrasound, CT and MRI. J Craniomaxillofac Surg 2000;28:319–24.

[16] Curtin HD, Ishwaran H, Mancuso AA, et al. Comparison of CT and MR imaging in the staging of neck metastases. Radiology 1998;207:123–30.

[17] van den Brekel MW. Lymph node metastases: CT and MRI. Eur J Radiol 2000;33:230–8.

[18] van den Brekel MW, Stel HV, Castelijns JA, et al. Cervical lymph node metastasis: assessment of radiologic criteria. Radiology 1990;177:379–84.

[19] King AD, Tse GM, Ahuja AT, et al. Necrosis in metastatic neck nodes: diagnostic accuracy of CT, MR imaging and US. Radiology 2004;230:720–6.

[20] King AD, Tse GM, Yuen EH, et al. Comparison of CT and MR imaging for the detection of extranodal neoplastic spread of metastatic neck nodes. Eur J Radiol 2004;52: 264–70.

[21] Yonetsu K, Sumi N, Izumi M, et al. Contribution of Doppler sonography blood flow information to the diagnosis of metastatic cervical nodes in patients with head and neck cancer: assessment in relation to anatomic levels of the neck. AJNR Am J Neuroradiol 2001;22: 163–9.

[22] Steinkamp HJ, Hosten N, Richter C, et al. Enlarged cervical lymph nodes at helical CT. Radiology 1994;191:795–8.

[23] Ishiawa M, Anzai Y. MR imaging of lymph nodes in the head and neck. Neuroimaging Clin N Am 2004;14:679–94.

[24] Sumi M, Ohki M, Nakamura T. Comparison of sonography and CT for differentiation of benign from malignant lymph nodes in patients with squamous cell carcinoma of the head and neck. AJR Am J Roentgenol 2001;176:1019–24.

[25] Steinkamp HJ, Cornehl M, Hosten N, et al. Cervical lymphadenopathy: ratio of long- to short-axis diameter as a predictor of malignancy. Br J Radiol 1995;68:266–70.

[26] Teknos TN, Rosenthal EL, Lee D, et al. Positron emission tomography in the evaluation of stage I and IV head and neck cancer. Head Neck 2001;23:1056–60.

[27] Schwartz DL, Rajendran J, Yueh B, et al. Staging of head and neck squamous cell carcinoma with extended-field FDG-PET. Arch Otolaryngol Head Neck Surg 2003;129:1173–8.

[28] Adams S, Baum RP, Stuckensen T, et al. Prospective comparison of 18F-FDG PET with conventional imaging modalities (CT, MRI, US) in lymph node staging of head and neck cancer. Eur J Nucl Med 1998;25:1255–60.

[29] Yen TC, Chang JT, Ng SH, et al. Staging of untreated squamous cell carcinoma of the buccal mucosa with 18F-FDG PET: comparison with head and neck CT/MRI and histopathology. J Nucl Med 2005;46:775–81.

[30] Brouer J, de Bree R, Comans EF, et al. Positron emission tomography using [18F]fluoro-deoxyglucose (FDG-PET) in the clinically negative neck: is it likely to be superior? Eur Arch Otorhinolaryngol 2004;261:479–83.

[31] Kataoka ML, Ueda H, Koyama T, et al. Contrast-enhanced volumetric interpolated breath-hold examination compared with spin-echo T1-weighted imaging of head and neck tumors. AJR Am J Roentgenol 2005;184:313–9.

[32] Escott EJ, Rao VM, Ko WD, et al. Comparison of dynamic contrast-enhanced gradient-echo and spin-echo sequences in MR of head and neck neoplasms. AJNR Am J Neuroradiol 1997;18:1411–9.

[33] Fischbein NJ, Noworolski SM, Henry RG, et al. Assessment of metastatic cervical lymph-adenopathy using dynamic contrast-enhanced MR imaging. AJNR Am J Neuroradiol 2003;24:301–11.

[34] Wang J, Takashima S, Takayama F, et al. Head and neck lesions: characterization with diffusion-weighted echo-planar imaging. Radiology 2001;220:621–30.

[35] Sumi M, Sakihama N, Sumi T, et al. Discrimination of metastatic cervical lymph nodes with diffusion-weighted MR imaging in patients with head and neck cancer. AJNR Am J Nero-radiol 2003;24:1627–34.

[36] Mack MG, Balzer JO, Straub R, et al. Superparamagnetic iron oxide-enhanced MR imaging of head and neck nodes. Radiology 2002;222:239–44.

[37] Sigl R, Vogl T, Casselman J, et al. Lymph node metastases from head and neck squamous cell carcinoma: MR imaging with ultrasmall superparamagnetic iron oxide particles (Sinerem MR)—results of a phase-III multicenter trial. Eur Radiol 2002;12:1104–13.

ELSEVIER
SAUNDERS

Otolaryngol Clin N Am
39 (2006) 319–329

OTOLARYNGOLOGIC
CLINICS
OF NORTH AMERICA

Dental Considerations in the Management of Head and Neck Cancer Patients

Eric H. Miller, DDS[a,b,*], Aubrey I. Quinn, BS[a]

[a]*School of Dentistry, University of Colorado Health Sciences Center, Denver, CO, USA*
[b]*University Hospital, Denver, CO, USA*

General principals

The most successful approach to managing the oral complications of therapy seen in head and neck cancer patients involves prevention and consultation. Pretreatment diagnosis and treatment is critical in preventing the serious sequelae of chemotherapy and head and neck radiation, and improving the patient's quality of life. A thorough oral examination is recommended, comprising an evaluation of the dentition and surrounding supportive periodontium, and a complete radiographic survey conducted as early in the course of treatment as possible. During this examination, hopeless and non-restorable teeth must be identified and removed before the induction of chemotherapy or the initiation of radiotherapy to minimize the risk for the development of complications, such as odontogenic facial abscesses and osteoradionecrosis. The early recognition of opportunistic infections, such as candidiasis or herpetic infections and their management also will improve the patient's overall health and outcome. The dental management of the head and neck cancer patient continues throughout the patient's course of treatment and afterwards with strict follow-up appointments to prevent post-treatment complications. Communication between the physician and dentist must be established and continued throughout the patient's course of treatment. The dentist must have an understanding of the patient's medical history, diagnosis, staging, and planned therapy to develop an

---

* Corresponding author. Hospital Dentistry Department of Diagnostic & Biological Sciences, University of Colorado at Denver and Health Sciences Center, School of Dentistry Mail Stop F844, P.O. Box 6508 Aurora, CO 80045.

E-mail address: Eric.Miller@uchsc.edu (E.H. Miller).

0030-6665/06/$ - see front matter © 2005 Elsevier Inc. All rights reserved.
doi:10.1016/j.otc.2005.11.011

appropriate treatment plan. For instance, the removal of teeth that lay outside a portal of radiation may prove unnecessary and of limited value in the patient's treatment. Additionally, performing oral surgery on an immunosupressed patient who has thrombocytopenia and neutropenia may result in serious complications not foreseen by the treating dentist. Detailed communication will aid greatly in preventing problems from arising.

The medical practitioner also should include a survey of the patient's oral cavity in the initial physical assessment of the patient. A general assessment may be performed quickly, noting the health of the gingival (soft tissues) and the state of the dentition. Are the soft tissues inflamed with evidence of bleeding or odor? Are there missing teeth? Are there loose teeth or mobile teeth? The findings may indicate the presence of periodontal disease. Swelling and painful, mobile teeth may signify a dentoalveolar abscess. A general understanding of dental disease will benefit the physician in their assessment of the patient.

The dentition is supported by the periodontium, comprising the surrounding alveolar bone, blood vessels, nerves, and connective tissues which surround the root surfaces of teeth. The connective tissue bundles which are termed the periodontal ligament (PDL) serve to attach the cementum of the root surface to the periosteum of the alveolar bone, thus securing the tooth in the alveolar "socket". In the healthy periodontum, little or no evidence of inflammation, bleeding, gingival recession or periodontal pocketing exists (Fig. 1). Early signs of periodontal disease may be manifested in gingivitis, in which the epithelialized gingival tissues are red, swollen, and inflamed (Fig. 2). Palpation and brushing or rinsing may evoke bleeding. When the underlying supportive tissues (alveolar bone, periosteum, and connective tissues) are comprised periodontitis or periodontal disease exists (Figs. 3 and 4).

The etiology and pathogenesis of periodontitis is complex, involving the bacterial flora of the oral cavity, the host defense mechanisms, and local factors, such as poor oral hygiene. Virulent bacteria, mainly gram-negative

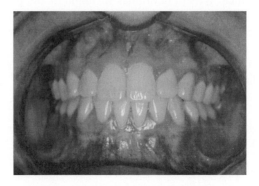

Fig. 1. Healthy dentition periodontium.

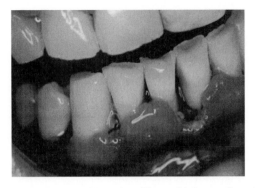

Fig. 2. Periodontitis. Note, blunted papillae and inflammation of gingiva.

rods and spirochettes, produces toxins which result in an immune-mediated response leading to the destruction of the periodontium. This destruction results in the clinical signs of tooth mobility, periodontal pocketing, suppuration, gingival recession, and swelling [1]. The examiner also may note the presence of an "anaerobic" odor. Most forms of periodontal disease are chronic and cyclic in nature, but radiotherapy and chemotherapy may cause an exacerbation of periodontitis. The management of periodontitis involves debridement and often the use of antibiotics. The goal of therapy is to remove the source of the inflammation and re-establish a normal oral flora. Further resective or reconstructive procedures may occur once the disease process has been controlled.

Dental caries or tooth decay affects the hard tissues—the enamel, underlying dentin, and the cementum of the root surface (Fig. 5). The process involves the acidic byproducts of bacterial metabolism decalcifying and destroying the calcified matrix of the hard structures of the tooth. Gram-negative bacteria is responsible, primarily, for the destruction seen in periodontitis, whereas gram-positive cocci, such as *streptococcus,* are responsible,

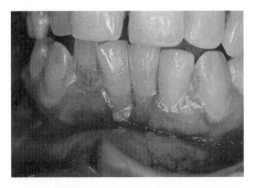

Fig. 3. Periodontitis manifested as localized recession.

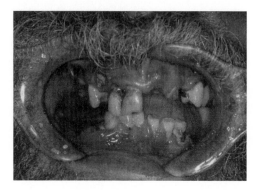

Fig. 4. Gross dental caries and periodontitis.

primarily, for dental caries. The physical signs of dental caries include discoloration and loss of tooth structure. Patients may complain of sensitivity to hot or cold. Dental decay may progress to the vital pulpal tissues of the tooth, leading to an increase in pain and sensitivity and often causing necrosis of the vital pulp and the formation of an abscess. The abscessed pulpal tissues may not present with symptoms if the vital nerve tissue within the dental pulp is necrotic, and abscesses may begin to extend to the surrounding alveolar bone. Abscesses involving the alveolar bone may spread rapidly to involve the fascial planes of the head and neck region, resulting in space infections or extensions beyond the head and neck region (Fig. 6) [2]. These infections may prove life-threatening and difficult to manage in the immunocompromised patient.

Active dental disease should be eliminated or at least minimized before the patient undergoes radiation therapy or chemotherapy. The presence of dental disease, either periodontitis or abscessed teeth, may cause significant problems in the management of the patient's head and neck cancer.

The dentist plays a critical role in the multidisciplinary approach to treating the head and neck cancer patient, providing a detailed pretreatment

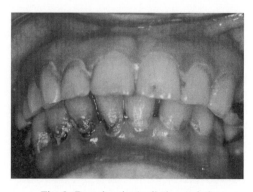

Fig. 5. Dental caries 'radiation caries'.

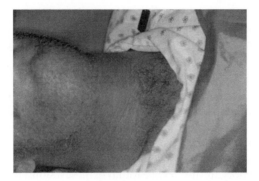

Fig. 6. Dental alveolar abscess resulting in submandibular and sublingual space infection.

evaluation of the patient, preparing the patient for treatment by eliminating all active dental disease and establishing improved oral health. The dental examination should include a detailed clinical examination with a full-mouth radiographic survey to ensure that all dental disease is revealed. Dental impressions should be taken in all patients who have teeth, for the fabrication of fluoride delivery trays and any maxillofacial prostheses, such as surgical obturators and oral appliances to aid in surgery and radiation therapy. Providing continued care of the patient following their treatment aids in preventing dental complications from occurring. Because that early staging and treatment is often the goal in managing head and neck cancer, it is imperative that a dental consultation be obtained early in the process. This accomplishes several objectives:

- The diagnosis of dental disease
- Early removal of nonrestorable teeth allowing for improved healing of the alveolar bone and periostium
- Early treatment of periodontal disease to improve overall oral health
- Implementation of preventative measures, such as fluoride use, and oral appliances designed to reduce treatment complications

Cases in which extraction of teeth is required, it is optimal to allow 14 to 21 days for healing of the alveolar bone before beginning radiation therapy [3]. This delay in beginning treatment often is not possible, underlying the importance of obtaining a dental consult early in the process.

Complications of head and neck radiotherapy

Osteoradionecrosis

The removal of nonrestorable or abscessed teeth in a timely manner lessens the risk for the patient developing osteoradionecrosis following radiotherapy. Osteoradionecrosis is seen as a chronic nonhealing lesion of bone that is caused primarily by an insult to nonvital bone. Irradiated bone presents with atrophic changes, including hypovascularity and hypocellularity, minimizing the regenerative capacity of the bone. These effects are dose related, with the risk for osteoradionecrosis increasing with higher dose volumes (> 50 cGy).

The mandible is involved more commonly than the maxilla because of the greater number of perimandibular tumors and limited blood supply (lack of ancillary vascularity) [4]. Trauma is the primary etiology of osteoradionecrosis, but it is also associated with periodontal disease, mucosal ulcerations, and dentoalveolar abscesses. Several cases occur spontaneously.

Although microorganisms may be found in these lesions, osteoradionecrosis is not believed commonly to be bacterial in origin, as in cases of osteomyelitis. Radiographic changes appear similar to the "moth-eaten" radiolucent patterns seen in osteomyelitis (Figs. 7 and 8). Sequestra or involucra may be seen clinically or radiographically. Progression of osteoradionecrosis (ORN) of the mandible may lead to pathologic fractures and extra-oral fistula complicating the successful management of this disease. Conservative debridement of sequestra combined with irrigation and peritreatment antibiotic therapy may be of value, but definitive surgical management should be combined with hyperbaric oxygen therapy.

Hyperbaric oxygen therapy enhances the diminished microvascular of irradiated bone and decreases tissue hypoxia, which often allows for replacement of nonvital bone. Improved oxygen tension also benefits osteoclastic and fibroblastic activity promoting the healing process [5].

It is recommended that post irradiation patients who require extraction of teeth or other procedures that traumatize irradiated bone undergo hyperbaric oxygen therapy before and after the procedure. A standard regimen of

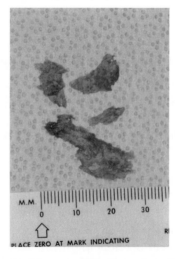

Fig. 7. Sequestrae removed from mandible of a patient with osteoradionecrosis.

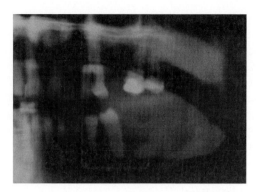

Fig. 8. Panorex of a patient with osteoradionecrosis of the right mandible.

20 pre-operative "dives" of 100% oxygen at 2.0 to 2.4 atmospheres for 90 to 120 minutes followed by 10 dives postoperatively is commonly followed [4]. Despite the relative effectiveness of hyperbaric oxygen therapy in the prevention and treatment of osteoradionecrosis, the benefit of preventative pre-irradiation treatment, such as extractions and periodontal treatment cannot be overemphasized when considering the risks and costs to the patient.

Xerostomia

Radiation therapy also may affect the salivary glands adversely, resulting in xerostomia. As with endothelium and bone, radiation damages acinar and ductal salivary gland cells, resulting in diminished or obliterated salivary flow. Saliva has digestive, antibacterial, and lubricating functions and the capability of acting as a pH buffer [6].

In post irradiated patients, there is a lower mean pH (5.48–6.05), resulting in a more acidic oral environment [7]. This environment leads to an increase in dental caries (especially affecting the less mineralized root surfaces) and oral infections. Patients also may have problems with speech, swallowing, and chewing food. Further complications of xerostomia may include esophagitis and nutritional insufficiencies.

Xerostomia is often difficult to manage. Patients should be encouraged to increase their water intake, reduce dietary sugars, and use fluoride treatments to minimize the risk for developing dental caries. Artificial saliva substitutes are available, offering lubrication and protection of the mucosa, and may aid in swallowing. Post irradiated patients require frequent maintenance visits and must be closely followed by their dentist.

In the xerostomic patient the prevention of dental caries is important. The lower pH and altered micoflora result in an increased risk for decay. The use of topical fluoride rinses and gels reduce the risk for dental caries. Numerous topical fluoride products are available by prescription and over the counter.

Methylcellulose based "saliva substitutes" are available also. System-
ically, xerostomia may be treated with pilocarpine and sialogogue, which stim-
ulates increased salivary production in patients who maintain some
measurable salivary flow. Pilocarpine 5 mg tablets may be given in a regimen
of 5 to 10 mg three times a day, not to exceed 30 mg daily. Cevimeline 30 mg
given in a dose of 30 to 60 mg three times daily has been useful in managing
xerostomia seen in Sjorgen's Syndrome [8]. These medications have potential adverse affects and interaction with other medications requiring consid-
eration before prescribing.

Opportunistic oral infections

Alterations in the oral environment that occur during and after radiation
and chemotherapy may result in oral infections by opportunistic organisms.
The diminished quality and quantity of saliva results in an altered pH, thus
allowing for the establishment of potential pathogens, such as *Candida albicans* and gram-negative rods and spirochetes. Normal saliva also has antibacterial properties that support the host immune response. The loss of
this salivary protection favors opportunistic infections.

Candida albicans is considered to be a normal commensal organism of
humans found primarily in the oropharynx and female genital tract. The
small cells reproduce by budding and have three morphologic forms: yeast,
pseudohyphae, and hyphae (filamentous) [9].

Clinically, oropharyngeal infections caused by *Candida* classically present
with whitish "patches" that rub away to reveal a raw bleeding mucosa surface. Candidal infections also may appear as a generalized redness to the
mucosal surfaces. Patients may complain of a "burning" sensation, altered
sense of taste, and nondescript pain. In the elderly and immunocompromised host, oral candidal infections may develop into oropharyngeal candidiasis, candidal esophagitis, and systemic infections.

The successful management of oral candidiasis relies on early diagnosis
and antifungal treatment. Various antifungal agents are available (Table 1).

Patients wearing dentures should remove the dentures and disinfect them
while receiving antifungal therapy. Patients whose treatment with topical
antifungal creams, ointments, powders and rinses fails should be placed immediately on systemic antifungals, such as ketoconazole and fluconazole. In
extreme cases, amphotericin B should be given intravenously.

Other opportunistic infections may occur during and after radiation therapy and chemoradiation. They include viral and bacterial infections, such as
herpetic infections and the establishment of periodontal pathogens that may
cause an exacerbation of periodontal disease.

Herpetic infections may be managed with antivirals, such as
acyclovir 200 mg five times daily for 10 days in initial and primary HSV

Table 1
Antifungal agents in the management of oral candidiasis

Agent	Dosage (adult)
Nystatin	
vaginal tablets 100,000u	1 tablet dissolved five times daily for 10–14 days
200,000u tablets (pastilles)	1 tablet qid for 10–14 days
100,000u/1 ml suspension	4–6 ml four times daily as rinse
Clotrimazole	
10 mg mycelex troches	1 tablet 5 times daily for 10–14 days
1% mycelex cream	apply to affected area four times daily
Ketoconazole	
200 mg tablets (Nizoral)	1 tablet daily for 10–14 days
Fluconazole	
50 and 100 mg tablets (Diflucan)	1 tablet daily for 10–14 days

Data from Langlais RP, Miller CS. Color atlas of common oral diseases. 2nd edition. Philadelphia: Lippincott, Williams & Wilkins; 1998. p. 152; and Oral health in cancer therapy. 1st edition. San Antonio: University of Texas; 2003. p. 25–6.

infections, and 200 to 400 mg five times daily in cases of recurrent HSV infections [10].

The management of periodontal disease was outlined earlier in this text and consists of debridement, antibiotic therapy (systemic and topical), or a combination.

Mucositis

The nonkeratinized epithelium of the oral mucosa is especially sensitive to radiation because of its rapid cellular proliferation, thus mucositis is a common and serious complication of radiation therapy and chemotherapy. Mucositis may develop early in the course of radiation therapy and often appears as generalized redness followed by pseudomembraneous ulceration [11]. The breakdown of the mucosa may be localized or generalized, and trauma often initiates the process.

The management of mucositis consists of palliative care and protecting the mucosa. Palliation may involve the use of a topical anesthetic such as 2% viscous xylocaine or narcotics in severe cases. Many commercially available compounds have been used to alleviate the discomfort of mucositis. Pharmacies and hospitals often have mixtures of coating agents, anti-inflammatories, and topical anesthetics, such as KBX (bismuth subsalicylate, diphenhydramine hydrochloride, and xylocaine) (Table 2). Mucositis is generally a self-limiting condition that improves within 2 months after radiation therapy; however, it may persist in the immunocompromised patient. Adequate hydration and nutritional intake is critical in dealing with patients who experience severe mucositis.

Table 2
Common topical agents utilized for the treatment of mucositis

saline rinses	methyclellulose
sodium bicarbonate rinse	propylcellulose
dilute hydrogen peroxide (1:4 to 1:10)	dyclonine HCI
kaopectate (kaolin-pectin)	xylocaine HCI
aluminum hydroxide	benzocaine HCI
magnesium hydroxide	diphenhydramine HCI

Data from Oral health in cancer therapy. 1st edition. San Antonio: University of Texas, 2003. p. 25–6; and Langlais RP, Miller CS. Color atlas of common oral diseases. 2nd edition. Philadelphia: Lippincott, Williams & Wilkins; 1998. p. 155.

Pre-surgical planning and prosthesis

For the patient facing surgical resection of the maxilla or mandible pre-surgical consultation is critical. The referring surgeon should communicate clearly with the dentist detailing the planned surgical procedure, including proposed surgical margins and postsurgical treatment (ie, radiation therapy).

Dental impressions should be taken at the initial visit before surgery if a prosthesis is planned to be placed immediately following surgery. In the event that a prosthesis is to be placed sometime after surgery, pre-operative dental impressions are of great value as that postsurgical trismus may limit the patient's ability to undergo prosthetic treatment. A dental prosthesis may require 1 to 2 weeks for a dental laboratory to fabricate, thus illustrating the importance of obtaining a dental consult early. Dental impressions also may be used to fabricate fluoride delivery trays for patients who are planned for radiotherapy to minimize the risk for developing dental caries. These trays are used by the patient to deliver concentrated fluoride to the vulnerable surfaces of the teeth, which reduces the process of decalcification and decay in the post irradiated xerostomic patient. Appliances also may be fabricated to protect oral tissues from radiation and aid in the management of trismus.

Summary

The text has emphasized the need for a timely dental consult early in the process of the head and neck cancer patient's treatment. Nonrestorable diseased teeth should be removed before radiation and chemotherapy. The primary survey of the patient should include an examination of the oral cavity, noting the state of the dentition and periodontal tissues.

Complications commonly seen in patient's undergoing radiotherapy, such as xerostomia, mucositis, and trismus, may be reduced and, therefore, improve the patient's quality of life. Optimizing the patient's oral health benefits the patient's postsurgical and postirradiation course. The dental health care professional can serve an important role in the overall outcome of the patient's care.

References

[1] Rateitschak KH, Rateitschak EM, Wolf MF, Hassell TM. Periodontology. 2nd edition. NY: Thieme Medical Publishers, Inc.; 1989. p. 1–48, 73–92.

[2] Topazian RG, Goldberg MH. Oral & maxillofacial infections. Philadelphia: WB Saunders Company; 1994. p. 205–6.

[3] Oral health in cancer therapy. 1st edition. San Antonio: University of Texas; 2003. p. 20.

[4] Topazian RG, Goldberg MH. Oral & maxillofacial infections. Philadelphia: WB Saunders Company; 1994. p. 280–3.

[5] Marx R, Stern D. Oral and maxillofacial pathology: a rationale for diagnosis and treatment. Chicago: Quintessence Publishing Company; 2003. p. 386–94.

[6] Ganong WF. Review of medical physiology. 19th edition. Stanford (CA): Appleton and Lange; 1999. p. 467.

[7] Oral health in cancer therapy. 1st edition. San Antonio: University of Texas; 2003. p. 25–6.

[8] Oral health in cancer therapy. 1st edition. San Antonio: University of Texas; 2003. p. 27.

[9] Gorbach SL, Bartlett JG, Blacklow NR. Infectious diseases. Philadelphia: WB Saunders Company; 1992. p. 1887–8.

[10] Gorbach SL, Bartlett JG, Blacklow NR. Infectious diseases. Philadelphia: WB Saunders Company; 1992. p. 1687–9.

[11] Lynch MA, Brightman VJ, Greenberg MS. Burket's oral medicine, diagnosis, and treatment. 9th edition. Philadelphia: JB Lippincott Company; 1984. p. 225–7.

ELSEVIER
SAUNDERS

Otolaryngol Clin N Am
39 (2006) 331–348

OTOLARYNGOLOGIC
CLINICS
OF NORTH AMERICA

The Surgical Management of Oral Cancer

John P. Campana, MD*, Arlen D. Meyers, MD, MBA

*Department of Otolaryngology, B-205, University of Colorado Health Sciences Center,
4200 East 9th Avenue, Denver, CO 80262, USA*

Oral cancer is the sixth most common cancer in the world [1]. It accounts for about 4% of all cancers and 2% of cancer deaths worldwide. In the United States, Europe, and Australia it accounts for 0.6% to 5% of all cancers, but it accounts for up to 30% of cancers in India [2]. In the United States alone, there are about 20,780 new cases and 5190 deaths from oral cavity cancer patient per year [3]. The incidence is twice as high in men than in women. Incidence rates have been slowly decreasing since the late 1970s.

Risk factors for oral cancer are well known. Approximately 75% of oral cancers are associated with cigarette smoking [4]. Alcohol works synergistically with smoking [5]. If tobacco and alcohol avoidance could be achieved, many of these malignancies could be prevented. Immunosuppression in transplant [6] and HIV patients [7] is also known to be a risk factor for oral cancer. Chewing betel quid is thought to account for the high rate of oral cancer in India [2,8]. Chewing tobacco certainly induces mucosal changes, which can be premalignant and can occur as early as 1 week after starting to chew [9]. The risk of developing cancer as the result of chewing tobacco, however, is less than that for smoking and may not be as great as was thought historically [10,11]. Tobacco use in all forms should be discouraged. Alcohol intake should be modest.

Anatomy, lymph node drainage, and staging

The oral cavity involves the mucosal lip anteriorly to the junction of the hard and soft palates superiorly and to the circumvallate papillae inferiorly. The subsites of the oral cavity are as follows [12]:

---

* Corresponding author.
E-mail address: John.Campana@uchsc.edu (J.P. Campana).

0030-6665/06/$ - see front matter © 2005 Elsevier Inc. All rights reserved.
doi:10.1016/j.otc.2005.11.005

Mucosal lip from the junction of the skin–vermillion border
Buccal mucosa
Lower alveolar ridge
Retromolar trigone
Upper alveolar ridge
Hard palate
Floor of the mouth
Oral anterior two thirds of the tongue

Lymph node drainage and nodal metastases tend to move in a predictable fashion. The first-echelon drainage of the oral cavity malignancies tends to go to the facial, submental, submandibular, and jugulodigastric nodes (zones I, II, and III). The second-echelon nodes include the parotid and lower remaining jugular and posterior triangle nodes (zones IV and V) [12,13]. Cancers at or near the midline metastasize bilaterally.

Management of suspicious lesions

Noonan and Kabani [14] recently wrote an excellent summary on the management of suspicious oral cavity lesions. They stressed that the term "leukoplakia" (Greek for "white, flat area") is a clinical descriptor only. Biopsies of leukoplakia show significant abnormalities ranging from dysplasias to overt invasive carcinoma 20% of the time. Carcinoma in situ presents as a leukoplakic lesion about 45% of the time. Higher-risk areas of leukoplakia include the soft palate, floor of the mouth, and the lateral and ventral tongue. Proliferative verrucous leukoplakia is a higher-risk lesion and usually progresses to overt cancer. Erythroplakia (Greek for "red, flat area") has almost a 90% chance of being a carcinoma in situ or invasive carcinoma. In judging the risk of malignant transformation, diploid lesions have less malignant potential than aneuploid lesions. Patients who have aneuploid lesions have a high risk of developing malignancy in other areas of the oral cavity and should be followed closely. In erythroleukoplakia, a combination of both lesions can occur.

If technically feasible, a complete surgical excision of these lesions is recommended to obtain a definitive diagnosis and is especially desirable for the high-risk lesions mentioned previously. For low-risk lesions, however, many use CO_2 laser and other superficial destructive techniques such as cryotherapy. CO_2 laser may play a role in management. Van der Hem and colleagues [15] reported an 89% cure rate after vaporizing leukoplakias. They had about a 10% rate of recurrent leukoplakia and a 1% rate of squamous cell carcinoma developing after treatment.

Benign lesions such as lichen planus, drug reactions, contact reactions, Candidiasis, traumatic lesions, and frictional keratosis should be considered in the differential diagnosis. Routine histologic evaluation and extra tissue for immunofluorescence is required to secure these diagnoses [14]. When in doubt, overt excision is recommended. If CO_2 laser ablation is considered, aggressive biopsy should be done in the most suspicious areas first.

Patients with field cancerization and diffuse or multiple scattered leukoplakias, erythroplakias, carcinomas in situ, and superficial invasive cancers present difficult management problems. Because of the significant morbidity of radiation therapy, some advocate photodynamic therapy using photosensitizers and laser light. In a small study by Schweitzer [16], complete responses were achieved in 8 of 10 patients who had diffuse field cancerization of the oral cavity with follow-up from 6 months to 9 years.

Work-up and staging of oral cancer

If the patient is cooperative, essentially all cancers of the oral cavity are easily accessible for transoral biopsy using local anesthetic in the office. The clinician should estimate the tumor size and whether bony, facial skin, or deep tongue muscle invasion is present. Any clinically apparent or radiographically suspicious lymph nodes in the neck are usually considered regional metastases until proven otherwise. A fine-needle aspiration biopsy of a neck node is highly accurate [17]. In general, incisional or excisional biopsy of suspicious neck nodes should be avoided. If the node is deep, difficult to feel, or in an anatomically challenging area, ultrasound or CT guidance is useful. The presence or absence of lymph node metastasis is one of the most important prognostic indicators in head and neck cancer. If present, cervical node metastasis drops the cure rate by about 50% [13,18].

The extent of a work-up for metastatic cancer and synchronous primaries (head and neck, pulmonary, and esophageal) is controversial. The rate of synchronous primary cancers is between 2.6% and 15% [19,20]. Before CT scanning was available, clinical examination of the head and neck, a chest radiograph to look for metastasis, occasionally barium swallow studies, and panendoscopy were the methods used to stage patients before definitive treatment. With the arrival of CT and MRI scans, these technologies were rapidly integrated into the work-up of head and neck cancer because of increased diagnostic accuracy for the primary tumor, nodal metastasis, pulmonary metastasis, and second primaries [20,21]. Now, CT/positron emission tomography scan imaging is available in most communities. The authors believe use of these imaging modalities is becoming the standard of care for evaluating primary tumors, regional metastasis, distant metastasis, and second primaries in the work-up of head and neck cancer [22,23]. MRI is still of value for evaluating some specific tumors, such as those in which bone or perineural invasion is suspected [21], and in the evaluation of tongue malignancies, where MRI provides greater soft tissue detail than CT scanning. Most surgeons still consider routine panendoscopy appropriate [24], but its routine use may be more questionable than ever because of the improvements in imaging modalities. If a pulmonary or

mediastinal abnormality is found, consultation with the pulmonary or thoracic surgery services is appropriate.

Staging

The staging system for oral cancer is a relatively standard TNM system.
Box 1 gives the American Joint Committee on Cancer staging system, and
Box 2 outlines the American Joint Committee on Cancer stage groupings [12].

Multidisciplinary decision making regarding treatment

Following diagnosis and staging, patients are presented to a multidisciplinary head and neck tumor board. If the tumor is a simple, small T1
N0 M0 cancer of the lateral oral tongue, and surgery only is the recommended therapy, the patient may be followed by the head and neck surgery team
only. Patients who have more advanced-stage cancer are usually seen and
managed by radiation oncology, medical oncology, and the head and
neck surgery services as a team. If radiation therapy is involved (either external beam using intensity-modulated radiotherapy techniques or brachytherapy), comprehensive dental care is extremely important to avoid
complications such as osteoradionecrosis [25]. Also, almost all patients receiving chemoradiation therapy directed at areas where severe mucositis is
likely or a significant operation from which dysphagia is expected will
need a percutaneous endoscopic gastrostomy feeding tube [26].

General comments on the paradigm shift in the treatment of head and neck cancer and its application to oral cancer

The authors generally manage T1/T2 cancers of the oral cavity surgically
to avoid the severe side effects of radiation to the mouth. More advanced
lesions are treated with combination therapy. There has been a paradigm
shift in the treatment of many advanced head and neck cancers [27]. T3/
T4 tumors traditionally were treated with resection and postoperative radiation. With or without obvious nodes, a neck dissection was usually done.
Now, the treatment of advanced head and neck cancer is changing. T3/T4
soft tissue–only cancers, with and without neck disease, now are most commonly treated with chemoradiation first and usually with a delayed, planned
neck dissection if there is clinically or radiographically persistent neck disease [28]. Surgery is also used for salvage at the primary site if there is residual or recurrent disease.

In the oral cavity this paradigm shift of primary chemoradiation with surgery for salvage often does not apply very well. Tumors of the oral
cavity frequently abut or overtly invade the maxilla or the mandible.
In these patients, primary chemoradiation can result in exposed bone, osteoradionecrosis, pathologic fractures, and infected, necrotic fields [29].
Therefore, the primary treatment of advanced oral cancers with close or

Box 1. American Joint Committee on Cancer TNM definitions for oral cancers

Primary tumor (T)
- TX: Primary tumor cannot be assessed
- T0: No evidence of primary tumor
- Tis: Carcinoma in situ
- T1: Tumor 2 cm or less in greatest dimension
- T2: Tumor larger than 2 cm but 4 cm or less in greatest dimension
- T3: Tumor larger than 4 cm in greatest dimension
- T4: (lip) Tumor invades through cortical bone, inferior alveolar nerve, floor of the mouth, or skin of face (ie, chin or nose)
- T4a: (oral cavity) Tumor invades adjacent structures (eg, through cortical bone, into deep [extrinsic] muscle of tongue [genioglossus, hyoglossus, palatoglossus, and styloglossus], maxillary sinus, and skin of face)
- T4b: Tumor invades masticator space, pterygoid plates, or skull base or encases internal carotid artery (Note: Superficial erosion alone of bone/tooth socket by gingival primary is not sufficient to classify a tumor as T4.)

Regional lymph nodes (N)
- NX: Regional lymph nodes cannot be assessed
- N0: No regional lymph node metastasis
- N1: Metastasis in a single ipsilateral lymph node, 3 cm or less in greatest dimension
- N2: Metastasis in a single ipsilateral lymph node, larger than 3 cm but 6 or less cm in greatest dimension; in multiple ipsilateral lymph nodes, 6 cm or less in greatest dimension; in bilateral or contralateral lymph nodes, 6 cm or less in greatest dimension
- N2a: Metastasis in a single ipsilateral lymph node larger than 3 cm but 6 cm or less in greatest dimension
- N2b: Metastasis in multiple ipsilateral lymph nodes, 6 cm or less in greatest dimension
- N2c: Metastasis in bilateral or contralateral lymph nodes, 6 cm or less in greatest dimension
- N3: Metastasis in a lymph node larger than 6 cm in greatest dimension

Distant metastasis (M)
- MX: Distant metastasis cannot be assessed
- M0: No distant metastasis
- M1: Distant metastasis

Box 2. American Joint Committee on oral cancer stage groupings

Stage 0
- Tis, N0, M0

Stage I
- T1, N0, M0

Stage II
- T2, N0, M0

Stage III
- T3, N0, M0
- T1, N1, M0
- T2, N1, M0
- T3, N1, M0

Stage IVA
- T4a, N0, M0
- T4a, N1, M0
- T1, N2, M0
- T2, N2, M0
- T3, N2, M0
- T4a, N2, M0

Stage IVB
- Any T, N3, M0
- T4b, any N, M0

Stage IVC
- Any T, any N, M1

Initial staging is done clinically and radiographically. Final staging is based on histology if surgery is performed.

---

overt bone involvement still usually involves surgery first, often with composite resection and more complicated reconstructions, followed by chemoradiation.

General issues related to surgery of the oral cavity

Preoperative

Malnutrition and low albumin levels are significant preoperative risk factors [30]. Nutritional supplementation, even for a short time before surgery, can sometimes help aid healing [31]. Preanesthesia testing and medical evaluations are done as necessary for the patient. An in-depth consultation including the appropriate surgical risks should be done. Although deep venous thrombosis and pulmonary embolus are rare complications in head and neck surgery patients, sequential compression stockings are usually placed if the operation will last longer than an hour or two [32]. Some surgeons also use low-dose unfractionated heparin or low-molecular-weight heparin. Prophylactic antibiotics, with some anaerobic coverage, are given in clean, contaminated cases [33].

In the operating room

The patient is placed on the operating table in a reversed fashion so the head is at the foot of the table. The patient is appropriately padded to prevent stasis ulcers and put in reverse Trendelenberg's position to minimize head edema. The authors place a urinary catheter for operations lasting longer than 4 hours. The patient is anesthetized through either a nasotracheal tube or a tracheotomy. Intraoperatively, the authors use frozen-section margin control. This technique can be done even on bone marrow if the surgery involves composite resection, although it is less reliable in such cases [34].

Neck dissection

Neck dissection is a frequent part of the treatment of oral cancer. The presence of neck nodes in early-stage malignancies of the head and neck can cut survival rates by half and is an extremely important prognostic indicator [13,18]. The patterns of nodal spread in the neck are relatively predictable [13]. The overall occult metastatic rate from oral cavity cancers to the neck is 34% [13]. It has been found that staging selective neck dissection is as good as radical neck dissection in the N0 neck [35]. Modified radical neck dissection (saving the spinal accessory nerve) is as good as radical neck dissection when there is obvious disease [36]. Some groups advocate the use of selective neck dissection even when there is known neck disease and report outcomes equivalent to radical neck dissection [37]. Jalisi [38] recently did a comprehensive review regarding the management of the clinically negative neck in early oral cavity cancer and concluded that neck observation is appropriate only for T1/T2 mucosal lip carcinomas, T1/T2 oral tongue carcinomas less than 4 mm thick, and T1/T2 floor of the mouth cancers that are 1.5 mm thick or less. Contralateral nodes should be treated if the tumor is midline, bilateral, or approaches or crosses the midline. The clinically negative neck should be treated if the risk of occult lymph node metastasis is greater than 20% [39]. It does not seem to matter if this treatment is elective neck dissection or elective radiation therapy: they are equivalent treatments in the N0 neck [40]. The neck should always be treated in patients who have larger T3 and T4 cancers because of the high incidence of nodal metastasis [41]. Sentinel node biopsy is not the standard of care for head and neck malignancies [42]. Multiple trials are in place to study this issue.

Reconstruction

The simplest technique that restores the highest level of cosmetic form and practical function is the best reconstruction. For the oral cavity, this sequence of techniques progresses as follows:

Granulation and secondary intent
Primary closure
Split-thickness skin grafts or allogenic dermal grafts
Local advancement flaps
Regional flaps
Pedicled myocutaneous flaps
Free flaps

Mandibular plating systems are also frequently required for fixation of the mandible after mandibulotomies or labiomandibulotomies, which are occasionally done to improve access for excision and reconstruction. Reconstruction plates are also used to reinforce rim mandibulectomies or to span mandibular gaps, usually in conjunction with pedicled or free flaps.

Osseointegrated implants are occasionally used in the maxilla to help anchor palatal prosthetics and dentures. The same is true for neomandibles that are constructed using free flaps after composite resections of the oral cavity. Osseointegrated implants can provide a more stable platform for lower dentures and maxillary prostheses, improving the patient's appearance and ability to chew [43,44]. Unfortunately, their use in an irradiated field can sometimes lead to loss of implants and precipitate osteoradionecrosis [45,46]. Hyperbaric oxygen may help retain implants [47], but not all surgeons placing these implants think hyperbaric oxygen is necessary [48].

Site-specific surgical management in the oral cavity

Mucosal lip from the junction of the skin–vermillion border

Small lesions of the upper and lower mucosal lip can be excised and allowed to granulate or be closed primarily. As the defect size increases, mucosal advancement flaps or split-thickness skin grafts can be used. If the cancer becomes large enough to require a through-and-through lip defect, wedge excisions with primary closure or local lip advancement flaps are used. These local flaps include bilateral advancement flaps, unilateral and bilateral melolabial flaps, Abbe-Estlander flaps, Gilles fan flaps, Karapandzic flaps, Bernard-Burow flaps, and their modifications [49]. In irradiated fields with larger residual cancers or with very large lip cancers, where the viability or utility of local flaps is questionable, many surgeons reconstruct a large lip defect with a radial forearm free flap or other similar soft tissue free flap [50]. If the lip cancer is large enough to include a composite mandibular resection, composite free flap reconstruction is also usually used. Twin free flaps are sometimes necessary [51]. When used to reconstruct the lower lip, the free flaps usually need to be suspended with a fascial sling, palmaris longus sling, or temporalis muscle sling to help the patient avoid drooling [50,51]. Because their bulk and propensity to sag leads to greater problems with oral incompetence, regional myocutaneous flaps are usually not favored for lip reconstruction.

Buccal mucosa

Small lesions of the buccal mucosa can also be excised and allowed to granulate or be closed primarily. Mucosal advancement flaps or split-thickness skin grafts can be used as the size of the defect increases. Larger and deeper buccal deficits can be filled with a temporalis muscle flap [52] or temporoparietal fascial flap [53], with or without a split-thickness skin graft or a temporal fasciocutaneous island flap [54]. If the cancer becomes large enough to require a full-thickness through-and-through cheek defect, the complexity of the reconstruction obviously increases. For smaller full-thickness cheek defects, one of the temporal flaps mentioned previously can be used internally to seal the oral cavity and provide bulk to the cheek. If the temporalis muscle flap is used, it may also provide an element of reanimation if the zygomaticus major and minor muscles have been taken. External coverage with a cervicofacial advancement flap completes the reconstruction. As the defect increases in size, a pedicled flap option would be a pectoralis myocutaneous flap with the skin paddle rotated either internally or externally and with a split-thickness skin graft to the exposed muscle [55]. A simple microvascular option for reconstruction would include a radial forearm flap with a de-epithelialized portion that would allow the flap to be folded on itself for internal and external lining [56] or a two-paddle subscapular system flap that would provide separate skin paddles for internal and external closure. A more complicated microvascular option would be the same two-paddle subscapular system flap transferred with part of the serratus anterior muscle and its long thoracic nerve. If the proximal facial nerve branch to the midface muscle is available for neurorrhaphy, this more complicated flap would provide closure and reanimation on a single vascular pedicle [57]. If the mandible is taken in conjunction with the buccal mucosa only, and the overlying skin is intact, most microvascular surgeons would consider a fibula osteocutaneous free flap as the first choice [58]. If the mandible is sacrificed, and there is a through-and-through full-thickness cheek defect, there are multiple options [59], including composite radial forearm free flap, fibula free flap, and double free flaps. Another excellent option may be a composite subscapular system free flap involving bone, two skin paddles, with or without serratus muscle and the long thoracic nerve, on a single vascular pedicle [57,60].

Lower alveolar ridge

The limited submucosal tissue over the alveolus and around the tooth sockets leads to early mandibular erosion by cancers in this region. Superficial erosion of mandibular bone or the tooth socket is not sufficient to classify a tumor as a T4, however. Occasionally, very early cancers of the lower alveolus may be excised without a bone margin and closed with local mucosal advancement flaps, but most early cancers of the alveolar ridge usually require a marginal mandibulectomy. A marginal mandibulectomy is considered appropriate and oncologically sound as long as the malignancy does not involve the alveolar canal [61–65]. Reconstruction plates are sometimes used to reinforce rim mandibulectomies. For cancers that invade deeper into the mandible, segmental resection is required. Reconstruction is similar to that described in the previous section regarding the use of free flaps to close segmental mandibular defects [44].

Retromolar trigone

Cancers of the retromolar trigone also tend to erode the mandible early because of the limited amount of submucosal tissue in the area. A rim mandibulectomy involving the anterior ramus of the mandible is sometimes possible. Masseter muscle flaps [66], palatal island flaps based on the greater palatine vessels [67], and temporalis flaps [68] are reconstructive options using local tissue to reconstruct the soft tissue of the retromolar trigone. If the surgeon is uncertain whether a segmental resection of the lateral mandible will be required, a lateral mandibulotomy can be made to increase visualization of the tumor site. A lateral mandibulotomy sacrifices the inferior alveolar nerve but avoids a facial incision. Also, if the surgeon needs to take part of the mandible to obtain negative margins, a smaller mandibulectomy occurs than with the hemimandibulectomy that would be required if an anterior mandibulotomy were done. If the ramus is sacrificed in a segmental resection, short lateral defects of the mandible (< 5 cm) can usually be spanned by a reconstruction bar and a soft tissue flap, most commonly either a pedicled pectoralis myocutaneous flap or a radial forearm free flap [69–71]. Composite free flaps can also be used, especially if the mandibular gap is greater than 5 cm. Reconstruction bars are usually fitted with the holes drilled and screws placed before the bone cuts of a mandibulotomy or segmental resection are made. The bar is removed for the mandibulotomy or composite resection and then replaced using the same holes for the reconstruction. This technique helps maintain normal mandibular position and occlusion if the patient has teeth.

Upper alveolar ridge and hard palate

The upper alveolar ridge and hard palate are usually considered together because even early cancers of this area usually span the two subsites. As in the upper alveolus and retromolar trigone, there is limited submucosal tissue in these areas, and bone erosion can occur even with relatively early cancers. Temporalis flaps and palatal island flaps are local tissues that can be used to reconstruct smaller defects. For smaller upper alveolar ridge and hard palate malignancies, prosthetics can be a simple and highly functional method of reconstruction. Free flaps, often radial forearm flaps, can also be used effectively [72]. Larger defects in this area frequently require a combination of free flap and prosthetic reconstruction to attain a high level of function [73]. Rectus and subscapular system flaps are sometimes used for larger maxillary reconstructions, especially if the overlying facial skin is involved. Large regional pedicled flaps, such as pectoralis flaps, are not useful in this region because of their bulk and difficulty in reaching the area.

Floor of the mouth and oral anterior two thirds of the tongue

The floor of the mouth and anterior two thirds of the tongue are also considered together because the extirpative and reconstructive principles are similar. Small cancers of these areas can be excised and left to granulate. Small tongue excisions can be closed primarily. A split-thickness skin graft or allogenic dermal graft can be used to resurface larger defects in either the floor of the mouth or oral tongue.

Visualization of the floor of the mouth is easy in edentulous patients and obviously harder in those with teeth. If possible, most surgeons try to avoid an anterior labiomandibulotomy or a lateral mandibulotomy for access to the floor of the mouth, lingual gutter, and tongue. These approaches are appropriate, however, if they are required to get negative margins. A mandibular lingual release, dropping the floor of the mouth and tongue into the neck, is an alternative in some cases [74].

An anterior or median mandibulotomy is associated with a facial incision and some damage to the anatomic structures in the floor of the mouth but preserves the inferior alveolar neurovascular bundle. Midline and parasymphaseal incisions heal well and are cosmetically acceptable [75]. With the advent of reconstruction bars, the traditional stair-step mandibulotomy is probably not necessary. Some surgeons sacrifice a tooth and run the mandibulotomy through the socket of that tooth. Some surgeons try to run their cut between two teeth, hoping saving them both but possibly putting both at risk for loss. The bone cut is usually made lateral to the genioid tubercle to avoid disturbing the muscle insertion of the genioglossus. If mandibular invasion is encountered when an anterior mandibulotomy has been done, the patient is committed to a hemimandibulectomy and usually free flap reconstruction, because the defect length is so long. With a lateral mandibulotomy, the inferior alveolar nerve is sacrificed, but, a facial incision is avoided, and a smaller mandibulectomy occurs.

As the cancers enlarge, involving more of the tongue, floor of the mouth, and lingual gutter, a thin, pliable, reconstruction like the radial forearm free flap or lateral upper arm free flap is usually preferred to help maintain as much mobility as possible [76]. Many surgeons reinnervate radial forearm free flaps in this area, providing some useful sensation [77]. When the defects of the tongue and floor of the mouth become massive, involving most of the oral tongue, bulkier pedicled flaps (such as a large pectoralis) and free flaps (rectus, subscapular, and anterolateral thigh) are usually better [78]. These bulkier flaps fill the space in the oral cavity where the tongue used to be and passively help get food and fluids to the back of the throat to aid somewhat with the impaired swallowing. Sometimes palatal prostheses are added to occlude this oral cavity dead space further and aid in swallowing.

If the cancer involves the mandible, and a composite resection is required, composite free flap reconstruction is almost universally recommended for the anterior mandibular arch [44]. If the anterior mandible is not reconstructed, it leads to the infamous "Andy Gump" deformity, which gives the patient the appearance of having an extremely weak or no chin. Anteriorly, a reconstruction bar and soft tissue–only reconstruction usually leads to plate exposure, with the bar often coming straight through the chin skin.

Through-and-through defects of the tongue, floor of the mouth, mandible, and facial skin require a three-component closure: internal lining, bone, and external skin. The subscapular system can provide two skin paddles and vascularized bone on a single vascular pedicle [57] and can be an excellent option. Some surgeons prefer a two-flap reconstruction often involving a pedicled and free flap [79]. A fibula osteocutaneous flap with the anastomosis in one side of the neck to reconstruct a large bony defect and reline the anterior floor of the mouth and a pectoralis myocutaneous flap from the contralateral neck to fill the external skin defect would be one such plan, among many.

Surgical complications

Infection, bleeding, cranial nerve injuries, and chyle leaks from neck dissections, tracheal stenosis and pneumothorax from tracheotomy, peritonitis from percutaneous gastric feeding tube placement, free flap venous occlusion and failure, decubitus ulcers, deep venous thrombosis and pulmonary embolus from long surgery times, repeat surgeries, recurrence, and multiple other complications can occur [80]. Management of these issues is beyond the scope of this article. Considering the complexity of many of these cases, most patients do well, have few complications, and leave the hospital relatively quickly. As an example, cancer cases requiring free flap reconstruction are some of the most complicated cases done. Free flap survival rates are

frequently reported to be between 95% and 99% [81,82], and hospitaliza-
tions for patients who have free flap reconstructions are usually about
1 week [83].

Survival by stage

The overall 5-year survival rate for oral cavity cancer is 46% to 59%
[3,84,85] and has not improved significantly in several decades. Early diagnosis is critical in minimizing treatment morbidity and, possibly, improving survival. Survival rates are site specific but by TNM stage generally are [85–87]

Stage I: 53% to 90%
Stage II: 54% to 100%
Stage III: 37% to 71%
Stage IV: 15% to 50%

Racial minorities have a significantly worse prognosis than whites [88].

Locally recurrent disease and second primary metachronous cancers

Although follow-up protocols vary widely, patients who have head and
neck cancer treated at the University of Colorado Health Sciences Center
are seen usually seen monthly for the first year after treatment, every
2 months during the second year, every 3 months during the third year, every 4 months during the fourth year, and every 6 months in the fifth year.
Positron emission tomography/CT scans are used in high-risk patients at
4- to 6-month intervals for the first 2 to 3 years.

Local recurrence is emotionally devastating to the patients, who frequently
have already been through a stressful course of treatment, and is challenging
for the physicians involved. If a recurrence is deemed resectable, and radiation
with or without chemotherapy was used initially, the authors offer surgical salvage. If surgery was the initial treatment, repeat surgery is frequently offered,
usually followed by chemoradiation. Re-irradiation is appropriate in some
cases but is a highly morbid protocol and has limited use [89]. If an ipsilateral
or a contralateral metastatic lymph node becomes apparent in a previously
untreated neck, surgery or radiation therapy may be appropriate. If the recurrence is unresectable, treatment becomes palliative.

There is about a 2% rate of developing second primary cancers per year
after treatment of the initial head and neck cancer [90]. In this population
there is a 20% to 22% chance of developing a second metachronous primary
cancer 5 years or more from the time of treatment for the initial cancer
[91,92]. These metachronous cancers most commonly occur in the head
and neck, esophagus, and lungs. Continued tobacco and alcohol use increases the risk of a second primary cancer. Radiation therapy can increase
the risk of developing second primary cancers [93]. The survival rates for
second primary cancers are lower than those for the initial cancers [94].

Palliation

Patients who have unresectable or metastatic disease are treated pallia-tively. Palliation usually involves chemotherapy, radiation therapy, or both. Surgery is usually limited to tracheotomy and insertion of a percutane-ous endoscopic gastrostomy feeding tube. Occasionally local tumor hygiene procedures are done if it is thought they will improve the patient's overall quality of life. Chemotherapy or re-irradiation with chemotherapy is offered to some patients [95].

Summary

Oral cavity cancers represent an area of head and neck oncology with some unique and interesting management themes. In spite of a significant paradigm shift in the treatment of many head and neck cancers toward us-ing primary chemoradiation, this treatment is not frequently applied to the oral cavity. Small cancers of the oral cavity are usually managed by surgery alone. Larger cancers are usually treated with primary surgery followed by chemoradiation. Neck treatment is offered to patients who have a greater than 20% chance of having lymph node metastasis or who have neck disease at the time of presentation. Neck treatment may involve surgery, radiation therapy, or both. Reconstruction of surgical defects of the oral cavity runs the gamut of techniques from the most simple to the most complex three-dimensional microvascular composite flaps. A multidisciplinary setting with a tumor board and multiple supportive services provides the best care for patients who have advanced-stage cancers.

References

[1] Parkin SM, Laara E, Muir CS. Estimates of the worldwide frequency of sixteen major can-cers in 1980. Int J Cancer 1988;41(2):184–97.
[2] Nair UJ, Friesen M, Richard I, et al. Effect of lime composition on the formation of reactive oxygen species from the areca nut extract in vitro. Carcinogenesis 1990;11:2145–8.
[3] American Cancer Society. Cancer facts and figures 2005. Atlanta (GA): American Cancer Society; 2005. p. 4;15.
[4] Scully C, Porter S. Oral cancer. BMJ 2000;321(7253):97–100.
[5] Choi SY, Kahyo H. Effect of cigarette smoking and alcohol consumption in the etiology of cancer of the oral cavity, pharynx, and larynx. Int J Epidemiol 1991;20:878–85.
[6] Hasegawa W, Pond GR, Rifkind JT, et al. Long-term follow-up of secondary malignancies in adults after allogeneic bone marrow transplantation. Bone Marrow Transplant 2005; 35(1):51–5.
[7] Haigentz M Jr. Aerodigestive cancers in HIV infection. Curr Opin Oncol 2005;17(5):474–8.
[8] Chang MC, Chiang CP, Lin CL, et al. Cell-mediated immunity and head and neck cancer: with special emphasis on betel quid chewing habit. Oral Oncol 2005;41(8):757–75.
[9] Payne JB, Johnson GK, Reinhardt RA, et al. Histologic alterations following short-term smokeless tobacco exposure in humans. J Periodont Res 1998;35(5):274–9.
[10] Bouquot JE, Meckstroth RL. Oral cancer in a tobacco-chewing US population—no ap-parent increased incidence of mortality. Oral Surg Oral Med Oral Pathol 1998;86(6): 697–706.

[11] Rodu B, Cole P. Smokeless tobacco use and cancer of the upper respiratory tract. Oral Surg Oral Med Oral Pathol 2002;93(5):511–5.

[12] Greene FL, Page DL, Flemming ID, et al. Lip and oral cavity. In: American Joint Committee on Cancer staging manual. 6th edition. New York: Springer; 2002. p. 23–32.

[13] Shah JP. Patterns of cervical lymph node metastasis from squamous carcinomas of the upper aerodigestive tract. Am J Surg 1990;160(4):405–9.

[14] Noonan VL, Kabani S. Diagnosis and management of suspicious lesions of the oral cavity. Otolaryngol Clin North Am 2005;38:21–35.

[15] van der Hem PS, Nauta JM, van der Wal JE, et al. The results of CO2 laser surgery in patients with oral leukoplakia: a 25 year follow up. Oral Oncol 2005;41(1):31–7.

[16] Schweitzer VG. Photofrin-mediated photodynamic therapy for treatment of early stage oral cavity and laryngeal malignancies. Lasers Surg Med 2001;29(4):305–13.

[17] Layfield LJ. Fine-needle aspiration of the head and neck. Pathology (Phila) 1996;4(2): 409–38.

[18] Sanderson RJ, Ironside JA. Squamous cell carcinomas of the head and neck. BMJ 2002; 325(7368):822–7.

[19] Davidson J, Gilbert R, Irish J, et al. The role of panendoscopy in the management of mucosal head and neck malignancy-a prospective evaluation. Head Neck 2000;22(5):449–54 [discussion: 454–5].

[20] Houghton DJ, Hughes ML, Garvey C, et al. Role of chest CT scanning in the management of patients presenting with head and neck cancer. Head Neck 1998;20(7):614–8.

[21] Alberico RA, Husain SH, Sirotkin I. Imaging in head and neck oncology. Surg Oncol Clin N Am 2004;13(1):13–35.

[22] Goerres GW, von Schulthess GK, Steinert HC. Why most PET of lung and head-and-neck cancer will be PET/CT. J Nucl Med 2004;45(Suppl 1):66S–71S.

[23] Kutler DI, Wong RJ, Kraus DH. Functional imaging in head and neck cancer. Curr Oncol Rep 2005;7(2):137–44.

[24] Guardiola E, Pivot X, Dassonville O, et al. Is routine triple endoscopy for head and neck carcinoma patients necessary in light of a negative chest computed tomography scan? Cancer 2004;101(9):2028–33.

[25] Chambers MS, Garden AS, Kies MS, et al. Radiation-induced xerostomia in patients with head and neck cancer: pathogenesis, impact on quality of life, and management. Head Neck 2004;26(9):796–807.

[26] Lin HS, Ibrahim HZ, Kheng JW, et al. Percutaneous endoscopic gastrostomy: strategies for prevention and management of complications. Laryngoscope 2001;111(10):1847–52.

[27] Moyer JS, Wolf GT, Bradford CR. Current thoughts on the role of chemotherapy and radiation in advanced head and neck cancer. Curr Opin Otolaryngol Head Neck Surg 2004;12(2): 82–7.

[28] Kutler DI, Patel SG, Shah JP. The role of neck dissection following definitive chemoradiation. Oncology 2004;18(8):993–8 [Williston Park].

[29] Turner SL, Slevin NJ, Gupta NK, et al. Radical external beam radiotherapy for 333 squamous carcinomas of the oral cavity—evaluation of late morbidity and a watch policy for the clinically negative neck. Radiother Oncol 1996;41(1):21–9.

[30] van Bokhorst-de, van der Schueren MA, van Leeuwen PA, Sauerwein HP, et al. Assessment of malnutrition parameters in head and neck cancer and their relation to postoperative complications. Head Neck 1997;19(5):419–25.

[31] Hujala K, Sipila J, Pulkkinen J, et al. Early percutaneous endoscopic gastrostomy nutrition in head and neck cancer patients. Acta Otolaryngol 2004;124(7):847–50.

[32] Agnelli G. Prevention of venous thromboembolism in surgical patients. Circulation 2004; 110(24, Suppl 1):IV4–12.

[33] Johnson JT, Kachman K, Wagner RL, et al. Comparison of ampicillin/sulbactam versus clindamycin in the prevention of infection in patients undergoing head and neck surgery. Head Neck 1997;19(5):367–71.

[34] Forrest LA, Schuller DE, Karanfilov B, et al. Update on intraoperative analysis of mandibular margins. Am J Otolaryngol 1997;18(6):396–9.

[35] Spiro RH, Morgan GJ, Strong EW, et al. Supraomohyoid neck dissection. Am J Surg 1996; 172(6):650–3.

[36] Andersen PE, Shah JP, Cambronero E, et al. The role of comprehensive neck dissection with preservation of the spinal accessory nerve in the clinically positive neck. Am J Surg 1994; 168(5):499–502.

[37] Andersen PE, Warren F, Spiro J, et al. Results of selective neck dissection in management of the node-positive neck. Arch Otolaryngol Head Neck Surg 2002;128(10):1180–4.

[38] Jalisi S. Management of the clinically negative neck in early squamous cell carcinoma of the oral cavity. Otolaryngol Clin North Am 2005;38(1):37–46.

[39] Weiss MH, Harrison LB, Isaacs RS. Use of decision analysis in planning a management strategy for the stage N0 neck. Arch Otolaryngol Head Neck Surg 1994;120(7):699–702.

[40] Chow JM, Levin BC, Krivit JS, et al. Radiotherapy or surgery for subclinical cervical node metastases. Arch Otolaryngol Head Neck Surg 1989;115(8):981–4.

[41] Tankere F, Camproux A, Barry B, et al. Prognostic value of lymph node involvement in oral cancers: a study of 137 cases. Laryngoscope 2000;110(12):2061–5.

[42] Ross G, Shoaib T, Soutar DS, et al. The use of sentinel node biopsy to upstage the clinically N0 neck in head and neck cancer. Arch Otolaryngol Head Neck Surg 2002;128(11):1287–91.

[43] Foster RD, Anthony JP, Sharma A, et al. Vascularized bone flaps versus nonvascularized bone grafts for mandibular reconstruction: an outcome analysis of primary bony union and endosseous implant success. Head Neck 1999;21(1):66–71.

[44] Urken ML, Buchbinder D, Costantino PD, et al. Oromandibular reconstruction using microvascular composite flaps: report of 210 cases. Arch Otolaryngol Head Neck Surg 1998; 124(1):46–55.

[45] Nishimura RD, Roumanas E, Beumer J III, et al. Restoration of irradiated patients using osseointegrated implants: current perspectives. J Prosthet Dent 1998;79(6):641–7.

[46] Esser E, Wagner W. Dental implants following radical oral cancer surgery and adjuvant radiotherapy. Int J Oral Maxillofac Implants 1997;12(4):552–7.

[47] Larsen PE. Placement of dental implants in the irradiated mandible: a protocol involving adjunctive hyperbaric oxygen. J Oral Maxillofac Surg 1997;55(9):967–71.

[48] Andersson G, Andreasson L, Bjelkengren G. Oral implant rehabilitation in irradiated patients without adjunctive hyperbaric oxygen. Int J Oral Maxillofac Implants 1998;13(5): 647–54.

[49] Larrabee WF, Sherris DA. Lips and chin. In: Principles of facial reconstruction. Philadelphia: Lippincott-Raven; 1995. p. 170–219.

[50] Langstein HN, Robb GL. Lip and perioral reconstruction. Clin Plast Surg 2005;32(3): 431–45.

[51] Jeng SF, Kuo YR, Wei FC, et al. Reconstruction of extensive composite mandibular defects with large lip involvement by using double free flaps and fascia lata grafts for oral sphincters. Plast Reconstr Surg 2005;115(7):1830–6.

[52] Wong TY, Chung CH, Huang JS, et al. The inverted temporalis muscle flap for intraoral reconstruction: its rationale and the results of its application. J Oral Maxillofac Surg 2004; 62(6):667–75.

[53] Alonso del Hoyo J, Fernandez Sanroman J, Gil-Diez JL, et al. The temporalis muscle flap: an evaluation and review of 38 cases. J Oral Maxillofac Surg 1994;52(2):143–7.

[54] Lopez R, Dekeister C, Sleiman Z, et al. The temporal fasciocutaneous island flap for oncologic oral and facial reconstruction. J Oral Maxillofac Surg 2003;61(10):1150–5.

[55] Vartanian JG, Carvalho AL, Carvalho SM, et al. Pectoralis major and other myofascial/myocutaneous flaps in head and neck cancer reconstruction: experience with 437 cases at a single institution. Head Neck 2004;26(12):1018–23.

[56] Disa JJ, Liew S, Cordeiro PG. Soft-tissue reconstruction of the face using the folded/multiple skin island radial forearm free flap. Ann Plast Surg 2001;47(6):612–9.

[57] Sullivan MJ. Subscapular system. In: Urken ML, Cheney ML, Sullivan MJ, et al, editors. Atlas of regional and free flaps for head and neck reconstruction. New York: Raven; 1995. p. 213–6.

[58] Mehta RP, Deschler DG. Mandibular reconstruction in 2004: an analysis of different techniques. Curr Opin Otolaryngol Head Neck Surg 2004;12(4):288–93.

[59] Jeng SF, Kuo YR, Wei FC, et al. Reconstruction of concomitant lip and cheek through-and-through defects with combined free flap and an advancement flap from the remaining lip. Plast Reconstr Surg 2004;113(2):491–8.

[60] Deschler DG, Hayden RE. The optimum method for reconstruction of complex lateral oromandibular-cutaneous defects. Head Neck 2000;22(7):674–9.

[61] McGregor AD, MacDonald DG. Routes of entry of squamous cell carcinoma to the mandible. Head Neck Surg 1988;10(5):294–301.

[62] Ord RA, Sarmadi M, Papadimitrou J. A comparison of segmental and marginal bony resection for oral squamous cell carcinoma involving the mandible. J Oral Maxillofac Surg 1997; 55(5):470–7.

[63] Lam KH, Lam LK, Ho CM, et al. Mandibular invasion in carcinoma of the lower alveolus. Am J Otolaryngol 1999;20(5):267–72.

[64] Tei K, Totsuka Y, Iizuka T, et al. Marginal resection for carcinoma of the mandibular alveolus and gingiva where radiologically detected bone defects do not extend beyond the mandibular canal. J Oral Maxillofac Surg 2004;62(7):834–9.

[65] Wolff D, Hassfeld S, Hofele C. Influence of marginal and segmental mandibular resection on the survival rate in patients with squamous cell carcinoma of the inferior parts of the oral cavity. J Craniomaxillofac Surg 2004;32(5):318–23.

[66] Antoniades K, Lasaridis N, Vahtsevanos K, et al. Superiorly based and island masseter muscle flaps for repairing oropharyngeal defects. J Craniomaxillofac Surg 2005;33(5):334–9.

[67] Genden EM, Lee BB, Urken ML. The palatal island flap for reconstruction of palatal and retromolar trigone defects revisited. Arch Otolaryngol Head Neck Surg 2001;127(7):837–41.

[68] Thomson CJ, Allison RS. The temporalis muscle flap in intraoral reconstruction. Aust N Z J Surg 1997;67(12):878–82.

[69] Arden RL, Rachel JD, Marks SC, et al. Volume-length impact of lateral jaw resections on complication rates. Arch Otolaryngol Head Neck Surg 1999;125(1):68–72.

[70] Shpitzer T, Gullane PJ, Neligan PC, et al. The free vascularized flap and the flap plate options: comparative results of reconstruction of lateral mandibular defects. Laryngoscope 2000;110(12):2056–60.

[71] Head C, Alam D, Sercarz JA, et al. Microvascular flap reconstruction of the mandible: a comparison of bone grafts and bridging plates for restoration of mandibular continuity. Otolaryngol Head Neck Surg 2003;129(1):48–54.

[72] Genden EM, Wallace DI, Okay D, et al. Reconstruction of the hard palate using the radial forearm free flap: indications and outcomes. Head Neck 2004;26(9):808–14.

[73] Bernhart BJ, Huryn JM, Disa J, et al. Hard palate resection, microvascular reconstruction, and prosthetic restoration: a 14-year retrospective analysis. Head Neck 2003;25(8):671–80.

[74] Devine JC, Rogers SN, McNally D, et al. A comparison of aesthetic, functional and patient subjective outcomes following lip-split mandibulotomy and mandibular lingual releasing access procedures. Int J Oral Maxillofac Surg 2001;30(3):199–204.

[75] Dubner S, Spiro RH. Median mandibulotomy: a critical assessment. Head Neck 1991;13(5): 389–93.

[76] Hara I, Gellrich NC, Duker J, et al. Swallowing and speech function after intraoral soft tissue reconstruction with lateral upper arm free flap and radial forearm free flap. Br J Oral Maxillofac Surg 2003;41(3):161–9.

[77] Netscher D, Armenta AH, Meade RA, et al. Sensory recovery of innervated and non-innervated radial forearm free flaps: functional implications. J Reconstr Microsurg 2000;16(3):179–85.

[78] Kimata Y, Sakuraba M, Hishinuma S, et al. Analysis of the relations between the shape of the reconstructed tongue and postoperative functions after subtotal or total glossectomy. Laryngoscope 2003;113(5):905–9.

[79] Blackwell KE, Buchbinder D, Biller HF, et al. Reconstruction of massive defects in the head and neck: the role of simultaneous distant and regional flaps. Head Neck 1997;19(7):620–8.

[80] Johns ME. Complications in otolaryngology: head and neck surgery, vol. 2. Philadelphia: B.C. Decker; 1986.

[81] Chalian AA, Anderson TD, Weinstein GS, et al. Internal jugular vein versus external jugular vein anastomosis: implications for successful free tissue transfer. Head Neck 2001;23(6): 475–8.

[82] Genden EM, Rinaldo A, Suarez C, et al. Complications of free flap transfers for head and neck reconstruction following cancer resection. Oral Oncol 2004;40(10):979–84.

[83] Rosenthal E, Carroll W, Dobbs M, et al. Simplifying head and neck microvascular reconstruction. Head Neck 2004;26(11):930–6.

[84] Casiglia J, Woo SB. A comprehensive review of oral cancer. Gen Dent 2001;49(1):72–82.

[85] Pugliano FA, Piccirillo JF, Zequeira MR, et al. Clinical-severity staging system for oral cavity cancer: five-year survival rates. Otolaryngol Head Neck Surg 1999;120(1):38–45.

[86] Shah JP, Lydiatt WM. Buccal mucosa, alveolus, retromolar trigone, floor of mouth, hard palate, and tongue tumors. In: Thawley SE, Panje WR, Batsakis JG, et al, editors. Comprehensive management in head and neck tumors, vol. 1. 2nd edition. Philadelphia: WB Saunders; 1999. p. 686–94.

[87] de Cassia Braga Ribeiro K, Kowalski LP, Latorre Mdo R. Perioperative complications, co-morbidities, and survival in oral or oropharyngeal cancer. Arch Otolaryngol Head Neck Surg 2003;129(2):219–28.

[88] Shavers VL, Brown ML. Racial and ethnic disparities in the receipt of cancer treatment. J Natl Cancer Inst 2002;94(5):334–57.

[89] Kasperts N, Slotman B, Leemans CR, et al. A review on re-irradiation for recurrent and second primary head and neck cancer. Oral Oncol 2005;41(3):225–43.

[90] Dikshit RP, Boffetta P, Bouchardy C, et al. Risk factors for the development of second primary tumors among men after laryngeal and hypopharyngeal carcinoma. Cancer 2005; 103(11):2326–33.

[91] Leon X, Del Prado Venegas M, Orus C, et al. Metachronous second primary tumours in the aerodigestive tract in patients with early stage head and neck squamous cell carcinomas. Eur Arch Otorhinolaryngol 2005;262(11):905–9.

[92] Schwartz LH, Ozsahin M, Zhang GN, et al. Synchronous and metachronous head and neck carcinomas. Cancer 1994;74(7):1933–8.

[93] Hashibe M, Ritz B, Le AD, et al. Radiotherapy for oral cancer as a risk factor for second primary cancers. Cancer Lett 2005;220(2):185–95.

[94] Bhattacharyya N, Nayak VK. Survival outcomes for second primary head and neck cancer: a matched analysis. Otolaryngol Head Neck Surg 2005;132(1):63–8.

[95] Hehr T, Classen J, Belka C, et al. Reirradiation alternating with docetaxel and cisplatin in inoperable recurrence of head-and-neck cancer: a prospective phase I/II trial. Int J Radiat Oncol Biol Phys 2005;61(5):1423–31.

ELSEVIER
SAUNDERS

Otolaryngol Clin N Am
39 (2006) 349–363

OTOLARYNGOLOGIC
CLINICS
OF NORTH AMERICA

Chemoprevention of squamous cell carcinoma of the oral cavity

Kevin S. Brown, MD[a],*,
Madeleine A. Kane, MD, PhD[b]

[a]Division of Hematology and Oncology, University of Colorado Health Sciences Center
and Denver Health Medical Center, Denver, CO, USA
[b]Division of Medical Oncology, University of Colorado Health Sciences Center
and Denver Veterans Affairs Medical Center, Denver, CO, USA

Squamous cell carcinoma of the oral cavity is the most common cancer of the head and neck region and is a major cause of morbidity and mortality worldwide. In the United States alone, over 28,000 cases are diagnosed each year [1]. Despite therapeutic advances in this disease, overall long-term survival remains less than 50%, and many of the long-term survivors are left with disfigurement and functional impairment as a result of surgery. Even in patients who are treated successfully with curative therapy, second primary tumors are a significant problem. Smoking and alcohol consumption are risk factors for the development of oral cavity squamous cell carcinoma (OCSCC). Betel quid chewing is a known risk factor in other parts of the world [2]. Human papilloma virus (HPV), particularly HPV type 16, may be an etiologic factor, especially among persons who do not smoke or drink alcohol [3,4]. Because of its easily-identifiable risk factors, and because premalignant lesions, such as leukoplakia, are often present in those who are destined to develop OCSCC, many disease prevention strategies have been evaluated in at-risk individuals. Prevention through the use of systemic medications, or chemoprevention, has been an extensively-studied strategy and continues to hold promise as a way of diminishing the morbidity and mortality associated with this disease.

* Corresponding author. Denver Health Medical Center, 660 Bannock Street, MC 4000, Denver, CO 80204.
   E-mail address: kevin.brown@dhha.org (K.S. Brown).

0030-6665/06/$ - see front matter © 2005 Elsevier Inc. All rights reserved.
doi:10.1016/j.otc.2005.11.010

Chemoprevention of other malignancies

Chemoprevention has been studied in several different malignancies, with some notable successes. Tamoxifen was shown in a large randomized prospective trial to significantly reduce the risk for breast cancer in high-risk women [5]. Nonsteroidal anti-inflammatory drugs have been associated with a decreased risk for colorectal cancer in epidemiologic studies [6]. The selective cyclooxygenase-2 (COX-2) inhibitor celecoxib has been shown to decrease several colonic polyps by 28% in persons with familial adenomatous polyposis [7].

Mechanisms of carcinogenesis

The development of OCSCC is a multistep process that involves changes related to specific genes, epigenetic events, and signal transduction within the cell (Fig. 1). Tobacco smoke contains agents that may act as mutagens [8]. Also, tobacco smoke extract has been shown to activate the epidermal growth factor receptor (EGFR) in vitro and EGFR activation has been shown, in turn, to increase the production of prostaglandins, including PGE2 which may act in a positive feedback fashion by increasing EGFR signal transduction [9]. Cyclin-D1 is frequently overexpressed in head and neck cancer, and increased cyclin-D1 activity is a downstream event triggered by EGFR activation [10]. Genetic alterations that are present early in the course of carcinogenesis are mutations or deletions of 3p and 9p. Telomerase activation also occurs early in carcinogenesis [11]. Mutations or deletions at 17p (involving the p53 tumor suppressor gene), and 13q and 18q generally are seen later in the process. Patients whose tumors contain HPV mRNA have a significantly lower rate of deletions of 3p, 9p, and 17p, suggesting an alternate molecular mechanism in these patients. The viral proteins E6 and E7 have been shown to cause deregulation of the cell cycle by inactivating p53 and

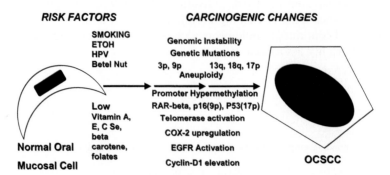

Fig. 1. Risk factors for development of oral cavity squamous cell cancer, and molecular events associated with progression to cancer.

retinoblastoma protein, which may be the mechanism of HPV-mediated carcinogenesis [3]. An important epigenetic event in the progression to cancer is the silencing of gene promoter regions through hypermethylation, which has been shown to affect the tumor suppressors p16, DAP-kinase, and E-cadherin [12,13]. Also, the gene for retinoic acid receptor-beta (RAR-beta) is silenced by methylation of its promoter [14]. In addition to deletions or mutations of individual genes, evidence exists demonstrating that numeric chromosomal imbalances, known as aneuploidy, may be a cause rather than a consequence of malignant transformation [15]. Aneuploidy may occur as a result of mutations in genes controlling chromosome segregation during mitosis and centrosome abnormalities [16,17].

Precancerous states

Oral leukoplakia, characterized by whitish mucosal plaques, is the most common identifiable precursor of OCSCC. Leukoplakia and erythroplakia, which is less prevalent but has a higher risk for progression to cancer, comprise the category of oral intraepithelial neoplasia (IEN). One study of 150 patients who present with leukoplakia followed for a mean of 103 months demonstrated a 24% risk for progression to OCSCC [18]. Many of the prevention studies performed to date have enrolled patients who present with oral leukoplakia and used regression of leukoplakia as a primary or secondary trial endpoint. IEN can be graded histologically according to the degree of dysplasia present, and dysplastic IEN has emerged as a distinct clinical entity with a high risk for progression to cancer. By adding ploidy analysis to the classification of these lesions, some investigators have defined aneuploid dysplastic IEN as a particularly high-risk precancerous lesion [10].

Local approaches to the management of IEN have been studied, with disappointing results. A study of 150 patients who present with dysplastic IEN showed that the success of resection in obtaining negative margins had no impact on the subsequent risk for developing OCSCC [19]. Another study similarly showed no overall benefit for negative resection margins but did show a benefit for molecularly confirmed negative resection margins in a subgroup of patients with high-risk mutations or loss of heterozygosity (LOH) patterns [20]. Other local approaches, such as radiation therapy and photodynamic therapy, remain investigational [10,21].

The difficulty of preventing progression of IEN to cancer with local therapies has been attributed to the multifocality, or "field cancerization" effect, of oral carcinogenesis. The field cancerization model, proposed by Slaughter and colleagues in 1953, hypothesized that exposure of the entire oral mucosa to carcinogens predisposed to the development of cancer at multiple sites within the oral cavity [22]. Recently, it has been shown by genetic analysis that cancers developing at distant sites within the oral cavity often are derived from the same initial clone [23]. The multifocality of the oral carcinogenesis process makes it difficult to interrupt the progression to cancer through the surgical removal of a premalignant lesion.

Chemopreventive agents

Many agents have been evaluated as possible chemopreventive therapies. Vitamins and minerals including vitamin A and other retinoids, beta-carotene, vitamin E, vitamin C, folates, and selenium have been studied. Herbal treatments have generated interest recently. Molecularly targeted approaches have included cyclooxygenase-2 (COX-2) inhibitors, EGFR inhibitors, and adenovirus vectors.

Vitamin A and other retinoids

Vitamin A and its derivatives, known collectively as the retinoids, have been some of the most extensively studied agents for the chemoprevention of OCSCC and head and neck cancer in general. Much has been learned from trials of these agents with regards to mechanisms of carcinogenesis and potential pathways of cancer prevention.

Observational studies provided some rationale for clinical chemoprevention trials using retinoids. An early case-control study showed significantly lower serum vitamin A levels in head and neck cancer patients than in healthy controls [24]. Another case-control study comparing head and neck cancer patients with and without second primary tumors found lower serum levels of vitamin A and vitamin E in patients with a second primary tumor than in those without [25].

In 1986, Hong and colleagues published a randomized, placebo-controlled trial of high-dose 13-cis-retinoic acid (isotretinoin) in the treatment of oral leukoplakia [26]. In this study, 44 patients were randomized to high-dose isotretinoin (1–2 mg per kg body weight daily for 3 months) or placebo. Sixty-seven percent of the patients in the treatment arm experienced a major decrease in the size of their lesions compared with 10% of patients in the placebo arm ($P = 0.0002$). Pathologic response as determined by resolution of dysplasia was seen in 54% versus 10% of patients ($P = 0.01$). Cheilitis, facial erythema, and skin dryness frequently were noted adverse events. Pathologic relapse occurred in 9 of 16 patients within 3 months of the end of the treatment period. This study was seen as proof of the feasibility of oral cancer chemoprevention, although the toxicity of the regimen and the short duration of the responses were clearly major problems. Subsequent studies of tissue from patients before treatment who exhibited high-dose isotretinoin showed decreased levels of RAR-beta messenger RNA in those who exhibited premalignant lesions versus normal controls, whereas expression of other retinoic acid receptor isoforms was not different between groups [27]. Levels of RAR-beta mRNA then increased after treatment with high-dose isotretinoin in 18 of 22 patients who had clinical response as compared with 8 of 17 patients who did not respond ($P = 0.04$). Other mechanisms for the activity of vitamin A have been postulated, including induction of intracellular cyclin D1 proteolysis and resultant lower intracellular cyclin D1 levels [28]. Another randomized study of moderately high-dose isotretinoin (50 to 100 mg per square meter) versus placebo in patients definitively treated for cancers of the larynx, pharynx, or oral cavity, failed to show a decrease in risk for tumor recurrence but did show a lower rate of development of second primary tumors in the treatment arm (24% versus 4%, $P = 0.005$) [29].

Because of concerns about the high rate of early relapses seen with a short course of high-dose isotretinoin, a subsequent trial in patients who present with leukolplakia evaluated an induction regimen of high-dose isotretinoin (1.5 mg/kg/d) for 3 months followed by randomization to maintenance therapy with beta-carotene (30 mg/d) or low-dose isotretinoin (0.5 mg/kg/d) for 9 months in patients who showed a response or stable disease with the initial 3-month treatment [30]. Fifty-five percent of patients responded to the induction phase of therapy. After randomization, 92% of patients in the low-dose isotretinoin arm versus 45% in the beta-carotene arm maintained their response or showed an additional degree of response ($P < 0.001$). Toxicity was significant still, particularly in the isotretinoin-only arm.

Other retinoid studies could not duplicate the beneficial effect of high-dose isotretinoin in preventing second primary tumors. The European Organization for Research and Treatment of Cancer (EORTC) performed a randomized, placebo-controlled trial of vitamin A (90 mg/d for 1 year followed by 45 mg/d for 1 year) alone compared with the antioxidant compound N-acetylcysteine alone for 2 years versus the combination of the two drugs for 2 years, in patients definitively treated for head and neck cancer or lung cancer [31]. This study showed no benefit for any of the intervention arms versus the placebo arm in overall survival, event-free survival, or second primary tumors. A total of 2592 patients were enrolled. A second, smaller European study involving 316 patients evaluated etretinate, a second-generation synthetic retinoid, versus placebo among patients definitively treated for oral cavity and oropharynx cancer [32]. This study did not show a benefit for etretinate in overall survival, disease-free survival, or development of second primary tumors.

Concerns were raised regarding potential harmful effects of vitamin A, and beta-carotene, among smokers by the Beta-Carotene and Retinol Efficacy Trial (CARET), published in 1996 [33]. Treated subjects received 7.5 mg (25,000 international units [IU]) of vitamin A along with 30 mg of beta-carotene daily. This study was designed as a randomized placebo-controlled primary lung cancer prevention trial, and enrolled 18,314 smokers, former smokers, and workers exposed to asbestos. The study showed a significantly higher risk for death from any cause, death from lung cancer, and death from cardiovascular disease in the treatment arm. Also, a randomized study of 25,000 units of vitamin A daily versus placebo demonstrated

3% higher total cholesterol and 1% lower HDL cholesterol levels among patients taking vitamin A [34].

Although toxicity concerns helped to somewhat dampen the enthusiasm surrounding vitamin A, some studies have continued. A small, Australian study randomized 151 patients definitively treated for head and neck cancer to high-dose isotretinoin (1 mg/kg/d), moderate-dose isotretinoin (0.5 mg/kg/d) or placebo. No difference was seen in the incidence of tumor recurrence, disease-free survival, or development of second primary tumors [35].

Some preclinical data, and clinical data in other tumor types, has suggested a possible benefit for combining retinoids with interferon-alpha [36–40]. A single-arm study of biochemoprevention in patients who present with premalignant lesions of the oral cavity or larynx using high-dose isotretinoin (80 mg/m^2/d), alpha-tocopherol (1200 IU/d) and interferon-alpha (3 million units/m^2 twice weekly) for 12 months showed some activity in laryngeal lesions (9 of 17 patients who demonstrated partial response, 3 who demonstrated complete response) but minimal activity in oral cavity lesions (4 of 10 patients who demonstrated partial response, no complete responses seen) [41]. A single-arm study of a somewhat lower dose of isotretinoin (50 mg/m^2/d) and a higher dose of interferon-alpha (3 million units/m^2 three times weekly) along with alpha-tocopherol 1200 mg daily for 12 months was performed in the adjuvant setting following definitive local therapy [42]. This study showed disease-free survival rates of 89%, 78%, and 74% at 1, 3, and 5 years, respectively. No second primary tumor development was seen. Based on these results, which compare favorably with historical controls, a randomized, placebo-controlled study is being conducted in the adjuvant setting.

Flavonoids

Flavonoids are a large group of low molecular weight polyphenolic phytochemicals found in all vascular plants. They are of interest because of their potentially beneficial role in the prevention of cancers and cardiovascular diseases, which is attributable to their antioxidant properties.

Studies of nutrient levels in the blood have suggested that deficiencies in carotenoids and vitamin E are associated with increased risk for oral and pharyngeal cancers. For example, a large case-control study with a cohort of 25,802 adults in Washington County, Maryland, found that serum levels of all carotenoids, including beta-carotene, were substantially lower in individuals who developed oral cancer, and decreased cancer risk was observed with higher levels. Low levels of alpha-tocopherol were associated with increased cancer risk also, but higher levels of gamma-tocopherol and selenium also were associated with increased risk [43]. However, oral mucosal tissue levels of carotenoids, retinoids, and tocopherols from chronic alcoholics who had oral cavity cancer compared with nonalcoholic controls who did not have cancer showed no significant differences in carotenoids or tocopherols; retinoids were more often detected in the mucosal tissue from the alcoholics [44].

A case-control study of micronutrient ingestion was conducted in 754 oral and pharyngeal cancer patients in Italy and Switzerland compared with 1775 control subjects with no history of cancer. Analysis of the results obtained using a validated food-frequency questionnaire observed odds ratios for carotene 0.61, vitamin E 0.74, vitamin C 0.63, folic acid 0.61, niacin 0.62 and vitamin B6 0.59; all were greater than one standard deviation below 1.0 [45].

A small single-arm study of 24 patients who presented with leukoplakia showed a complete plus partial response rate of 71% to a regimen of beta-carotene 30 mg daily for 3 months, followed by an additional 3 months of treatment in responding patients, with no significant toxicity reported [46]. A randomized, placebo-controlled trial that enrolled 264 patients who had definitively-treated oral cavity, pharyngeal, or laryngeal cancer showed no benefit of 50 mg of beta-carotene daily in overall survival, local recurrences, or development of second primary tumors [47].

The Physicians' Health Study, a long-term randomized placebo-controlled study of 22,071 male physicians in the United States showed no benefit nor harm for taking beta-carotene 50 mg on alternating days in overall survival, incidence of lung cancer, number of cancer deaths, or death from cardiovascular disease [48]. In contrast to the CARET trial noted above, however, only 11% of subjects were current smokers and 39% were former smokers at the beginning of this study, so these results did not alleviate concern regarding possible harmful effects of beta-carotene in smokers.

A randomized, double-blind, placebo-controlled primary prevention trial was performed in Finland to determine whether daily supplementation with alpha-tocopherol, beta-carotene, or both would reduce the incidence of lung cancer and other cancers. A total of 29,133 male smokers 50 to 69 years of age from southwestern Finland were randomly assigned to one of four regimens: alpha-tocopherol (50 mg/d) alone, beta-carotene (20 mg/d) alone, alpha-tocopherol and beta-carotene, or placebo. Follow-up continued for 5 to 8 years. No reduction in the incidence of lung cancer or other cancers was observed in any of the groups given supplementation [49].

Vitamin E

The term vitamin E describes a family of eight antioxidants, four tocopherols (alpha-, beta-, gamma-, and delta-) and four tocotrienols (also alpha-, beta-, gamma-, and delta-). Alpha-tocopherol is the only form of vitamin E that is actively maintained in the human body and its main function appears to be that of an antioxidant.

Studies using the hamster buccal pouch dimethyl benzanthracine (DMBA) model reported inhibitory effects of systemic alpha-tocopherol on tumor formation [50–52]. Lower serum levels of vitamin E in humans have been associated with increased risk for oral cancer as above [43]. A population-based case-control study of a variety of vitamin and mineral supplements found that vitamin E was the only supplement consistently associated with a lower risk for oral and pharyngeal cancers after controlling for tobacco, alcohol, and other supplement use. The odds ratio for vitamin E "ever users" was 0.5 [53]. Dietary antioxidant intake also has been studied using dietary recall methodology in patients treated for early-stage oral cavity cancer in comparison with historical controls. Cancer patients had a lower mean daily intake of fruits and vegetables and antioxidant nutrients (vitamins A, C, E and total carotenes) than age- and gender-matched historical controls, suggesting an association with oral cavity cancer risk [54]. A phase II study in patients who presented with oral leukoplakia administered alpha-tocopherol 400 IU twice daily for 24 weeks. In 43 patients who completed the planned treatment, 46% showed clinical responses and 21% showed histologic responses suggesting efficacy of vitamin E in reversal of these premalignant lesions [55].

Recent results of a large multicenter, double-blind, randomized, placebo-controlled chemoprevention trial for patients treated with radiation therapy for stage I or II squamous cell carcinoma of the head and neck have shown no benefit from vitamin E. A total of 540 patients were randomized to receive beta-carotene (30 mg/d) plus alpha tocopherol (400 IU daily) or placebo [56]. Beta-carotene supplementation was discontinued after the first 156 patients were enrolled because of ethical concerns, given toxicity results of other studies. After a median follow-up of 52 months, 113 second primary cancers and 119 recurrences were diagnosed. During the supplementation period, those receiving vitamin E had a higher rate of second primary cancers than those receiving placebo (hazards ratio [HR] = 2.88) but had a lower rate after supplementation was discontinued (HR = 0.41). Similar results were seen with recurrences (HR = 1.86 while on treatment; HR = 0.71 after discontinuation of treatment). The proportion of patients free of second primary cancers after 8 years was similar in the treated and placebo groups. Investigators concluded there were unexpected adverse effects on occurrence of second primary malignancies and cancer-free survival.

Vitamin C

Vitamin C, also known as ascorbic acid, is a water-soluble vitamin. Vitamin C is required for the synthesis of collagen, the neurotransmitter norepinephrine, and carnitine, and it is involved in the metabolism of cholesterol to bile acids. Vitamin C is also a highly effective antioxidant and can protect against damage by free radicals and reactive oxygen species.

Vitamin C supplementation reduced the incidence of squamous cell carcinomas of the skin in hairless mice exposed to ultraviolet radiation, suggesting a chemoprotective effect against cancer [57]. Higher concentrations of vitamin C induced apoptotic cell death in various tumor cell lines, including oral squamous cell carcinoma and salivary gland tumor cell lines, possibly by way of its prooxidant action. The apoptosis-inducing activity of ascorbate is stimulated by $Cu2+$, lignin and ion chelator, and inhibited by catalase, $Fe3+$, $Co2+$, and saliva. On the other hand, at lower concentrations, ascorbic acid displays an antioxidant property, preventing stress or antitumor agent-induced apoptosis [58]. In studies of human dietary nutrients, serum levels of nutrients, or vitamin C supplementation, chemopreventive effects have been less clear.

Folates

Folate coenzymes mediate the transfer of one-carbon units in various reactions critical to the metabolism of nucleic acids and amino acids. Nutritional studies have observed that diets high in fresh vegetables are associated with a lower incidence of squamous cell carcinoma in multiple sites in the upper aerodigestive tract, suggesting a protective effect of folates [59]. Mean folate levels in the blood of 42 squamous cell head and neck cancer patients were significantly lower than smoking or nonsmoking controls (5.8 ± 2.1 ng/ml versus 9.1 ± 2.7 ng/ml and 9.7 ± 2.2 ng/ml, respectively) [60]. Serum folate levels were significantly lower and homocysteine levels significantly higher in a group of 144 squamous cell cancer of the head and neck patients and 40 patients who present with laryngeal leukoplakia compared with 90 smoking or 120 nonsmoking controls [61]. A folate insufficiency status seems to be distinct from the conventional definition of folate deficiency in which DNA methylation patterns are altered [62]. Polymorphisms of enzymes that catalyze the single-carbon transfer reactions to provide the chemically relevant species of reduced folates may be impacted by folate sufficiency status. A more sensitive analysis of folate sufficiency, therefore, may uncover folate imbalances that result in aberrant DNA methylation patterns, which in turn predispose to biochemical changes leading to neoplasms. Folate deficiency predisposes to catastrophic neural tube defects in human fetuses that have certain methylenetetrahydrofolate reductase polymorphisms. These defects are prevented by folate supplementation during gestation [63]. Certain defined polymorphisms of the thymidylate synthetase $3'$ untranslated region have been reported to be associated with a decreased risk for squamous cell carcinoma of the head and neck (OR [odds ratio] $= 0.60$) and particularly oral cancer (OR $= 0.26$) [64]. Altered one-carbon transfer reactions essential to a balanced pool of nucleotide bases may result in misincorporation of bases into DNA, leading to increased strand breaks and global DNA hypomethylation. A hypothesis of the role that folate insufficiency and resulting imbalance in intracellular one-carbon transfer reactions may play in carcinogenesis of squamous cell carcinoma of the head and neck has been published [65].

Selenium

Selenium is a trace element that is essential in small amounts but can be toxic in larger amounts. Humans and animals require selenium for the function of several selenium-dependent enzymes, also known as selenoproteins.

Adequate selenium levels have been postulated to be chemopreventive. Age-adjusted death rates for cancer at most head and neck sites are lower in states where soil and forage crops contain higher levels of selenium. Erythrocyte selenium levels and erythrocyte and tissue levels of the selenium-dependent antioxidant enzyme glutathione peroxidase were lower in 50 patients who have untreated oral cavity or oropharyngeal cancers compared with age-matched controls; plasma selenium levels were higher in patients, however [66]. A case-control study of oral cancer cases versus controls found an OR of 1.4 for low selenium levels in nail tissue; OR was 1.9 for men but 0.6 for women. In patients 20 to 39 years of age, however, the OR was 16.4 for low selenium levels [67]. The impact of the selenium compounds selenodiglutathione (SDG) and 1,4-phenylenebis(methylene)selenocyanate (p-XSC) on normal human mucosal cells and human oral squamous carcinoma cells in primary culture was investigated. SDG induced significantly higher levels of apoptosis in SCCs than in normal cells, both compounds induced Fas ligand to an extent that correlated with degree of apoptosis, and both induced JNK and p38 kinase, and ERK 1 and 2. JNK induction seemed to be the most important for induction of apoptosis in studies using specific inhibitors, including dominant negative JNK [68]. In the F344 rat tongue cancer model (4-nitroquinolone-1-oxide, 4-NQO), development of squamous cell carcinoma of the tongue was reduced from 47% in control rats to 0% in rats treated with p-XSC [69].

Herbal treatments

Animal models that suggested a chemopreventive effect of the algae, Spirulina fusiformis [70], led to investigation into its impact on prevention or reversal of leukoplakia in humans. S. fusiformis (1g orally daily) or placebo was administered to pan tobacco chewers in India. After 12 months of daily treatment, complete regression of oral leukoplakia lesions was observed in 45% of those receiving the algae but in no controls. Serum beta-carotene and retinol levels were not different between groups [71].

Animal studies with the DMBA hamster cheek pouch model reported that the addition of black raspberries (5% or 10% lyophilized material added to diet for 2 weeks before DMBA treatment and for 10 weeks after) resulted in a significant reduction in the number of tumors observed compared with controls [72].

Molecularly-targeted approaches

Epidermal growth factor (EGFR) is known to be overexpressed in several epithelial tumors and in 80% to 100% of oral cavity cancerous and precancerous lesions [73,74]. COX-2, which is involved in the synthesis of prostaglandins, also has been found in increased amounts in various tumor types and premalignant lesions and wild-type but not mutant, p53 has been shown to inhibit COX-2 transcription in vitro [75]. Evidence exists demonstrating that prostaglandins produced by COX-2 activity are often involved in carcinogenesis, and prostaglandin E2 has been shown to activate EGFR with resultant stimulation of cell proliferation [76–78]. As noted above, the COX-2 inhibitor celecoxib was shown to decrease several colonic polyps in those with familial adenomatous polyposis. Preclinical evidence exists of increased activity of the combination of an EGFR inhibitor and a COX-2 inhibitor versus either agent alone in the suppression of tumor formation [79]. A randomized trial of the EGFR inhibitor EKB-569 alone, celecoxib (400 mg twice daily) alone, the combination of the two drugs or placebo in patients who presented with aneuploid dysplastic oral leukoplakia is being planned in Norway, Sweden, Denmark, and Finland [10]. Diagnoses of aneuploid dysplastic IEN are recorded in the national tumor registries of these countries. Despite the concern about an increase in cardiovascular events among patients taking COX-2 inhibitors, this particular patient population is at extremely high risk for developing OCSCC and, therefore, could potentially be a group where the benefit of oral cancer chemoprevention would outweigh the slightly increased cardiovascular risk associated with celecoxib.

ONYX-015 is an adenovirus vector that selectively replicates in and is selectively cytotoxic to cells that lack p53 protein [80,81]. This vector carries an inactivating mutation in the gene encoding the E1B 55-kd protein, which normally binds to and inactivates p53. In cells without p53 function, replication of a virus lacking the E1B 55-kd protein can proceed, whereas replication is inhibited in cells with normal p53 function. Therefore, ONYX-015 can cause, preferentially, lysis of p53-deficient cells. A nonrandomized trial evaluating three different doses of ONYX-015-laden mouthwash in patients who presented with oral IEN showed histologic resolution of dysplasia in 7 (37%) of 19 patients and an improvement of the severity of dysplasia in one additional patient [82]. Most of these responses were transient. The treatment was well-tolerated. A correlation was seen between normalization of p53 protein expression and histologic response, but similar correlations were not seen with cyclin D1 expression. Further trials of ONYX-015 are ongoing.

Summary

Squamous cell carcinoma of the oral cavity has long been seen as an attractive candidate for chemoprevention strategies. Because of the poor outcomes associated with the disease, the presence of identifiable premalignant lesions, and the failure of local preventive therapies, such as surgery, many investigators have hoped to find an effective chemopreventive compound. Initial enthusiasm surrounding high-dose retinoids gave way to concerns regarding toxicity and short duration of response. Although many of the other agents discussed above have shown promise, as yet none have been proven safe and effective in large-scale randomized trials. Much has been learned, however, about the molecular process of oral carcinogenesis from studies of these agents. Ongoing and future studies of chemopreventive agents in oral cancer hopefully will be able to exploit our expanding knowledge of these molecular pathways.

References

[1] Jemal A, Tiwari RC, Murray T, et al. Cancer Statistics, 2004. CA Cancer J Clin 2004;54(1): 8–29.
[2] Jeng JH, Chang MC, Hahn LJ. Role of areca nut in betal quid-associated chemical carcinogenesis: current awareness and future perspectives. Oral Oncol 2001;37(6):477–92.
[3] Braakhuis BJM, Snijders PJF, Keune W-JH, et al. Genetic patterns in head and neck cancers that contain or lack transcriptionally active human papillomavirus. J Natl Cancer Inst 2004; 96(13):998–1006.
[4] Mao L, Hong WK. How does human papillomavirus contribute to head and neck cancer development? J Natl Cancer Inst 2004;96(13):978–80.
[5] Fisher B, Costantino JP, Wickerham DL, et al. Tamoxifen for prevention of breast cancer: report of the National Surgical Adjuvant Breast and Bowel Project P-1 Study. J Natl Cancer Inst 1998;90(18):1361–70.
[6] Thun MJ, Namboodiri MM, Heath CW. Aspirin use and reduced risk of fatal colon cancer. N Engl J Med 1991;325(23):1593–6.
[7] Steinbach G, Lynch PM, Phillips RK, et al. The effect of celecoxib, a cyclooxygenase-2 inhibitor, in familial adenomatous polyposis. N Engl J Med 2000;342(26):1946–52.
[8] Jaloszynski P, Jaruga P, Olinski R, et al. Oxidative DNA base modifications and polycyclic aromatic hydrocarbon DNA adducts in squamous cell carcinoma of larynx. Free Radic Res 2003;37(3):231–40.
[9] Dannenberg AJ, Lippman SM, Mann JR, et al. Cyclooxygenase-2 and epidermal growth factor receptor: pharmacologic targets for chemoprevention. J Clin Oncol 2005;23(2):254–66.
[10] Lippman SM, Sudbo J, Hong WK. Oral cancer prevention and the evolution of molecular-targeted drug development. J Clin Oncol 2005;23(2):346–56.
[11] Mao L, Hong WK, Papadimitrakopoulou VA. Focus on head and neck cancer. Cancer Cell 2004;5:311–6.
[12] Hasegawa M, Nelson HH, Peters E, et al. Patterns of gene promoter methylation in squamous cell cancer of the head and neck. Oncogene 2002;21(27):4231–6.
[13] Herman JG, Baylin SB. Gene silencing in cancer in association with promoter hypermethylation. N Engl J Med 2003;349(21):2042–54.
[14] Youssef EM, Lotan D, Issa J-P, et al. Hypermethylation of the retinoic acid receptor-beta$_2$ gene in head and neck carcinogenesis. Clin Cancer Res 2004;10:1733–42.
[15] Sen S. Aneuploidy and cancer. Curr Opin Oncol 2000;12(1):82–8.
[16] Lengauer C, Kinzler KW, Vogelstein B. Genetic instabilities in human cancers. Nature 1998; 396(6712):643–9.
[17] Gardner RD, Burke DJ. The spindle checkpoint: two transitions, two pathways. Trends Cell Biol 2000;10(4):154–8.
[18] Sudbo J, Kildal W, Risberg B, et al. DNA content as a prognostic marker in patients with oral leukoplakia. N Engl J Med 2001;344(17):1270–8.

[19] Sudbo J, Lippman SM, Lee JJ, et al. The influence of resection and aneuploidy on mortality in oral leukoplakia. N Engl J Med 2004;350(14):1405–13.

[20] Zhang L, Poh CF, Lam WL, et al. Impact of localized treatment in reducing risk of progression of low-grade oral dysplasia: molecular evidence of incomplete resection. Oral Oncol 2001;37(6):505–12.

[21] Betz CS, Leunig A. Potential and limitations of fluorescence diagnosis and photodynamic therapy part 2: photodynamic therapy. HNO 2004;52(2):175–92.

[22] Slaughter DP, Southwick HW, Smejkal W. Field cancerization in oral stratified squamous epithelium: clinical implications of multicentric origin. Cancer 1953;6:963–8.

[23] Braakhuis BJ, Tabor MP, Kummer JA, et al. A genetic explanation of Slaughter's concept of field cancerization: evidence and clinical implications. Cancer Res 2003;63(8):1727–30.

[24] Murr G, Kostelic F, Donkic-Pavicic I, et al. Comparison of the vitamin A blood serum level in patients with head-neck cancer and healthy persons. HNO 1988;36(9):359–62.

[25] deVries N, Snow GB. Relationships of vitamins A and E and beta-carotene serum levels to head and neck cancer patients with and without second primary tumors. Eur Arch Otorhinolaryngol 1990;247(6):368–70.

[26] Hong WK, Endicott J, Itri LM, et al. 13-cis-retinoic acid in the treatment of oral leukoplakia. N Engl J Med 1986;315(24):1501–5.

[27] Lotan R, Xu X-C, Lippman SM, et al. Suppression of retinoic acid receptor-beta in premalignant oral lesions and its up-regulation by isotretinoin. N Engl J Med 1995;332(21):1405–11.

[28] Langenfeld J, Kiyokawa H, Sekula D, et al. Posttranslational regulation of cyclin D1 by retinoic acid: a chemoprevention mechanism. Proc Natl Acad Sci USA 1997;94(22): 12070–4.

[29] Hong WK, Lippman SM, Itri LM, et al. Prevention of second primary tumors with isotretinoin in squamous-cell carcinoma of the head and neck. N Engl J Med 1990;323(12): 795–801.

[30] Lippman SM, Batsakis JG, Toth BB, et al. Comparison of low-dose isotretinoin with beta-carotene to prevent oral carcinogenesis. N Engl J Med 1993;328(1):15–20.

[31] van Zandwijk N, Dalesio O, Pastorino U, et al. EUROSCAN, a randomized trial of vitamin A and N-acetylcysteine in patients with head and neck cancer or lung cancer. J Natl Cancer Inst 2000;92(12):977–86.

[32] Bolla M, Lefur R, Van JT, et al. Prevention of second primary tumours with etretinate in squamous cell carcinoma of the oral cavity and oropharynx. Results of a multicentric double-blind randomised study. Eur J Cancer 1994;30(6):767–72.

[33] Omenn GS, Goodman GE, Thornquist MD, et al. Effects of a combination of beta carotene and vitamin A on lung cancer and cardiovascular disease. N Engl J Med 1996;334(18): 1150–5.

[34] Cartmel B, Moon TE, Levine N. Effects of long-term intake of retinol on selected clinical and laboratory indexes. Am J Clin Nutr 1999;69(5):937–43.

[35] Perry CF, Stevens M, Rabie I, et al. Chemoprevention of head and neck cancer with retinoids: a negative result. Arch Otolaryngol Head Neck Surg 2005;131(3):198–203.

[36] Lingen MW, Polverini PJ, Bouck NP. Retinoic acid and interferon alpha act synergistically as antiangiogenic and antitumor agents against human head and neck squamous cell carcinoma. Cancer Res 1998;58(23):5551–8.

[37] Lindner DJ, Borden EC, Kalvakolanu DV. Synergistic antitumor effects of a combination of interferons and retinoic acid on human tumor cells in vitro and in vivo. Clin Cancer Res 1997;3(6):931–7.

[38] Lippman SM, Parkinson DR, Itri LM, et al. 13-cis-retinoic acid and interferon alpha-2a: effective combination therapy for advanced squamous cell carcinoma of the skin. J Natl Cancer Inst 1992;84(4):235–41.

[39] Lippman SM, Kavanagh JJ, Paredes-Espinoza MP, et al. 13-cis retinoic acid plus interferon-alpha 2a in locally advanced squamous cell carcinoma of the cervix. J Natl Cancer Inst 1993; 85(6):499–500.

[40] Motzer RJ, Schwartz L, Law TM, et al. Interferon alfa-2a and 13-cis-retinoic acid in renal cell carcinoma: antitumor activity in a phase II trial and interactions in vitro. J Clin Oncol 1995;13(8):1950–7.

[41] Shin DM, Mao L, Papadimitrakopoulou VM, et al. Biochemopreventive therapy for patients with premalignant lesions of the head and neck and p53 gene expression. J Natl Cancer Inst 2000;92(1):69–73.

[42] Shin DM, Richards TJ, Seixas-Silva JA, et al., Phase II trial of bioadjuvant therapy with interferon-alpha2a, 13-cis-retinoic acid, and alpha-tocopherol for locally advanced squamous cell carcinoma of the head and neck: long term follow-up [Abstract 1995]. In: Proceeding of the American Society of Clinical Oncology. Chicago: 2003. p. 496.

[43] Zheng W, Blot WJ, Diamond EL, et al. Serum micronutrients and the subsequent risk of oral and pharyngeal cancer. Cancer Res 1993;53(4):795–8.

[44] Leo MA, Seitz HK, Maier H, et al. Carotenoid, retinoid and vitamin E status of the oropharyngeal mucosa in the alcoholic. Alcohol Alcohol 1995;30(2):163–70.

[45] Negri E, Franceschi S, Bosetti C, et al. Selected micronutrients and oral and pharyngeal cancer. Int J Cancer 2000;86(1):122–7.

[46] Garewal HS, Meyskens FL Jr, Killen D, et al. Response of oral leukoplakia to beta-carotene. J Clin Oncol 1990;8(10):1715–20.

[47] Mayne ST, Cartmel B, Baum M, et al. Randomized trial of supplemental beta-carotene to prevent second head and neck cancer. Cancer Res 2001;61(4):1457–63.

[48] Hennekens CH, Buring JE, Manson JE, et al. Lack of effect of long-term supplementation with beta carotene on the incidence of malignant neoplasms and cardiovascular disease. N Engl J Med 1996;334(18):1145–9.

[49] The Alpha-Tocopherol, Beta Carotene Cancer Prevention Study Group. The effect of vitamin E and beta carotene on the incidence of lung cancer and other cancers in male smokers. N Engl J Med 1994;330(15):1029–35.

[50] Trickler D, Shklar G. Prevention by vitamin E of experimental oral carcinogenesis. J Natl Cancer Inst 1987;78(1):165–9.

[51] Calhoun KH, Stanley D, Stiernberg CM, et al. Vitamins A and E do protect against oral carcinomas. Arch Otolaryngol Head Neck Surg 1989;115(4):484–8.

[52] Sawant SS, Kandarkar SV. Role of vitamins C and E as chemopreventive agents in the hamster cheek pouch treated with the oral carcinogen DMBA. Oral Dis 2000;6:241–7.

[53] Gridley G, McLaughlin JK, Block G, et al. Vitamin supplement use and reduced risk of oral and pharyngeal cancer. Am J Epidemiol 1992;135(10):1083–92.

[54] Steward DL, Wiener F, Gleich LL, et al. Dietary antioxidant intake in patients at risk for secondary primary cancer. Laryngoscope 2003;113(9):1487–93.

[55] Benner SE, Winn RJ, Lippmann SM, et al. Regression of oral leukoplakia with alpha-tocopherol: a community clinical oncology program chemoprevention study. J Natl Cancer Inst 1993;85(1):44–7.

[56] Bairati I, Meyer F, Gelinas M, et al. Randomized trial of antioxidant vitamins to prevent acute adverse effects of radiation therapy in head and neck cancer patients. J Clin Oncol 2005;23(24):5805–13.

[57] Pauling L, Willoughby R, Reynolds R, et al. Int J Vitam Nutr Res Suppl 1982;23:53–82.

[58] Sakagami H, Satoh K, Hakeda Y, et al. Apoptosis-inducing activity of vitamin C and vitamin K. Cell Mol Biol 2000;46(1):129–43.

[59] Franceschi S, Bidoli E, Negri E, et al. Role of macronutrients, vitamins and minerals in the aetiology of squamous cell carcinoma of the oesophagus. Int J Cancer 2000;86(5):626–31.

[60] Almadori G, Bussu F, Galli J, et al. Serum folate and homocysteine levels in head and neck carcinoma. Cancer 2002;94(4):1006–11.

[61] Almadori G, Bussu F, Galli J, et al. Serum levels of folate, homocysteine and vitamin B12 in head and neck squamous cell carcinoma and in laryngeal leukoplakia. Cancer 2005;103(2):284–92.

[62] Rampersaud GC, Kauwell GPA, Hutson AD. Genomic DNA methylation decreases in response to moderate folate depletion in elderly women. Am J Nutr 2000;72: 998–1003.

[63] Werler MM, Shapiro S, Mitchell AA. Periconceptual folic acid exposure and risk of occurrent neural tube defects. JAMA 1993;269(10):1257–61.

[64] Zhang Z, Shi Q, Sturgis EM, et al. Thymidylate synthase 5′- and 3′- untranslated region polymorphisms associated with risk and progression of squamous cell carcinoma of the head and neck. Clin Cancer Res 2004;10(23):7903–10.

[65] Kane MA. The role of folates in squamous cell carcinoma of the head and neck. Cancer Detect Prev 2005;29(1):46–53.

[66] Goodwin WJ Jr, Lane HW, Bradford K, et al. Selenium and glutathione peroxidase levels in patients with epidermoid carcinoma of the oral cavity and oropharynx. Cancer 1983;51(1): 110–5.

[67] Negri E, Franceschi S, Bosetti C, et al. Selected micronutrients and oral and pharyngeal cancer. Int J Cancer 2000;86(1):122–7.

[68] Ghose A, Fleming J, El-Bayoumy K, et al. Enhanced sensitivity of human oral carcinomas to induction of apoptosis by selenium compounds: involvement of mitogen-activated kinase and Fas pathways. Cancer Res 2001;61(20):7479–87.

[69] Tanaka T, Makita H, Kawabata K, et al. 1,4-phenylenebis(methylene)selenocyanate exerts exceptional chemopreventive activity in rat tongue carcinogenesis. Cancer Res 1997;57: 3644–8.

[70] Schwartz J, Shklar G. Regression of experimental hamster cancer by beta carotene and algae extracts. J Oral Maxillofac Surg 1987;45:510–5.

[71] Mathew B, Sankaranarayanan R, Nair PP, et al. Evaluation of chemoprevention of oral cancer with Spirulina fusiformis. Nutr Cancer 1995;24:197–202.

[72] Casto BC, Kresty LA, Kraly CL, et al. Chemoprevention of oral cancer by black raspberries. Anticancer Res 2002;22:4005–15.

[73] Grandis JR, Tweardy DJ. Elevated levels of transforming growth factor alpha and epidermal growth factor receptor messenger RNA are early markers of carcinogenesis in head and neck cancer. Cancer Res 1993;53(15):3579–84.

[74] Shin DM, Ro JY, Hong WK, et al. Dysregulation of epidermal growth factor receptor expression in premalignant lesions during head and neck tumorigenesis. Cancer Res 1994; 54(12):3153–9.

[75] Subbaramaiah K, Altorki N, Chung WJ, et al. Inhibition of cyclooxygenase-2 gene expression by p53. J Biol Chem 1999;274(16):10911–5.

[76] Dannenberg AJ, Altorki NK, Boyle JO, et al. Cyclo-oxygenase 2: a pharmacological target for the prevention of cancer. Lancet Oncol 2001;2(9):544–51.

[77] Pai R, Soreghan B, Szabo IL, et al. Prostaglandin E2 transactivates EGF receptor: a novel mechanism for promoting colon cancer growth and gastrointestinal hypertrophy. Nat Med 2002;8(3):289–93.

[78] Buchanan FG, Wang D, Bargiacchi F, et al. Prostaglandin E2 regulates cell migration via the intracellular activation of the epidermal growth factor receptor. J Biol Chem 2003;278(37): 35451–7.

[79] Torrance CJ, Jackson PE, Montgomery E, et al. Combinatorial chemoprevention of intestinal neoplasia. Nat Med 2000;6(9):1024–8.

[80] Ries S, Korn WM. ONYX-015: mechanisms of action and clinical potential of a replication-selective adenovirus. Br J Cancer 2002;86(1):5–11.

[81] Heise C, Sampson-Johannes A, Williams A, et al. ONYX-015, an E1B gene-attenuated adenovirus, causes tumor-specific cytolysis and antitumoral efficacy that can be augmented by standard chemotherapeutic agents. Nat Med 1997;3(6):639–45.

[82] Rudin CM, Cohen EE, Papadimitrakopoulou VA, et al. An attenuated adenovirus, ONYX-015, as mouthwash therapy for premalignant oral dysplasia. J Clin Oncol 2003;21(24): 4546–52.

ELSEVIER
SAUNDERS

Otolaryngol Clin N Am
39 (2006) 365–380

OTOLARYNGOLOGIC
CLINICS
OF NORTH AMERICA

Current Radiation Therapy Management Issues in Oral Cavity Cancer

Ari Ballonoff, MD*, Changhu Chen, MD,
David Raben, MD

*Department of Radiation Oncology, University of Colorado Health Sciences Center,
Aurora, CO, USA*

Historically, cancers of the oral cavity have been managed surgically. Radiotherapy has emerged during the past two decades as a viable treatment modality either alone or in combination with surgery or chemotherapy. This article reviews the current role of radiation therapy and future management strategies in the treatment of head and neck cancers with an emphasis on carcinoma of the oral cavity.

Radiation is employed in three general situations: (1) as primary definitive therapy,(2) in the postoperative setting as an adjuvant therapy for patients who have high risk factors, and (3) as salvage therapy in the setting of failure after surgery or radiation. Issues relevant to this discussion include the use of concurrent chemoradiation, altered fractionation radiation, brachytherapy, and the incorporation of targeted therapies with radiation.

Because of the high recurrence rates in locally advanced disease treated with surgery or radiation, trial design over the past 10 years has incorporated concurrent chemoradiation therapy in an attempt to optimize outcomes. Recently, many trials have emerged showing a benefit of concurrent chemoradiation therapy versus radiation alone in both the definitive [1,2] and postoperative [3,4] settings in locally advanced disease. There is now evidence showing improved local control in patients who have locally advanced head and neck cancer receiving twice-daily radiation versus traditional once-daily radiation [5]. Additionally, more recent trials have explored the efficacy and tolerability of combining altered fractionation radiation with concurrent chemotherapy [6,7]. Despite these incremental improvements in the treatment of head and neck cancer, locally advanced disease continues

---

* Corresponding author. Department of Radiation Oncology, Campus Mail Stop F-706, P.O. Box 6510, Aurora, CO 80045.
  E-mail address: ari.ballonoff@uchsc.edu (A. Ballonoff).

0030-6665/06/$ - see front matter © 2005 Elsevier Inc. All rights reserved.
doi:10.1016/j.otc.2005.11.004

to have unacceptably high recurrence rates, and treatment can be associated with severe side effects. New targeted agents in combination with radiation or chemotherapy show promise in early phase I/II trials. These targeted agents act to perturb critical aspects of the cancer cell signaling pathway including the epidermal growth factor receptor (EGFR) cascade. Excitingly, a recent phase III trial has confirmed a survival benefit of anti–epidermal growth factor antibodies in combination with radiation for locally advanced head and neck cancer [8].

This review begins with a brief overview of the logistics of various radiation treatment modalities including external beam radiation, brachytherapy, and intraoral cones. Following is a review of the role of brachytherapy and external beam radiotherapy in the management of early stage disease. Treatment of locally advanced disease comprises the majority of the chapter, including the current state of knowledge regarding definitive chemoradiation, altered fractionation radiation, altered fractionation chemoradiation, and post-operative chemoradiation. Future directions, including the incorporation of targeted therapies into current therapeutic strategies conclude this article.

Radiation treatment modalities

Radiation can be delivered to the oral cavity in three general ways: by external beam radiation, interstitial implants, and intraoral cone therapy.

Most centers deliver radiation by a traditional external beam approach using linear accelerators that produce either photons or electrons. Before the radiation is delivered, a patient has a simulation appointment in the radiation oncology department. During simulation, a patient is positioned as during future treatments, usually with a special plastic mask that conforms to the facial features and skull. This mask is used to provide strict immobilization to achieve precise daily radiation treatments. A CT scan is then obtained using 3- to 5-mm thick slices through the head and neck region. The images are sent to treatment-planning computers, at which time the radiation oncologist defines the high-risk treatment volumes (the gross tumor and the involved or high-risk lymph node regions), low-risk treatment volumes that require less radiation dose (eg, uninvolved lymph nodes on the contralateral neck), and the structures to be spared (spinal cord, salivary glands). Dosimetrists then place fields to maximize dose to the treatment volume and minimize dose to critical structures. From the time of simulation, the radiation treatment plan usually takes 1 week to complete. The patient then returns and receives radiation, typically 5 days/week (Monday through Friday) or twice daily with at least a 6-hour interval between treatments to allow normal tissue recovery. Each treatment can last as little as 10 minutes (conventional radiation) or as long as 30 minutes (intensity-modulated radiation therapy), depending on the complexity of the plan.

The radiation oncologist sees the patient weekly to monitor the side effects and the patient's progress.

Interstitial implantation (brachytherapy) offers another way to deliver radiation to the oral cavity. Interstitial implantation has an advantage of steep fall-off of radiation dose in the surrounding tissue, thus sparing surrounding normal structures. Brachytherapy is usually done in conjunction with external beam radiation to boost the dose to the tumor, but it may be used alone in small T1/T2 N0 tumors. In conjunction with a head and neck surgeon, the radiation oncologist places either temporary catheters or permanent radioactive seeds directly into the visible tumor while the patient is under general anesthesia. In the case of catheter placement, the personnel in the radiation oncology department remotely load radioactive isotopes into the catheters for a specified period of time in a shielded room to prevent exposure of medical personnel to the radiation. After the treatment, the catheters are removed. Traditionally, low-dose-rate brachytherapy is used, but in recent years high-dose-rate brachytherapy has emerged as another useful option in head and neck brachytherapy. High-dose-rate brachytherapy delivers radiation treatment at a dose rate similar to that of external beam radiation; however, this type of brachytherapy generally involves the delivery, through robotics, of a high-activity radioactive source (Iridium-192, Ir^{192}) on the tip of a wire. This wire is automatically inserted rapidly into each temporary catheter for specified dwell times to deliver high-dose radiation in a few minutes.

Intraoral cones are specialized devices used to deliver external beam radiation. Like brachytherapy, they are used either before or after conventional external beam radiation to boost the dose to the tumor. The radiation oncologist chooses a cone that encompasses the visible tumor and attaches it to the x-ray unit. Low-energy radiation (125–250 kVp) is then delivered directly to the tumor while sparing most of the adjacent normal structures.

Radiation side effects and management

Radiation to the oral cavity can be very irritating to the patient. Radiation oncologists need to familiarize themselves with the potential acute toxicities and manage them so as not to delay treatment once radiation has started. During the first 1 to 2 weeks, patients usually notice minimal, if any, side effects other than a sensation of a dry mouth and changes in taste. Beginning in the third or fourth week, most patients notice increasing xerostomia with thickened saliva, mucositis, skin reaction, pain, and difficulty swallowing.

Xerostomia is a common side effect encountered by patients receiving radiation to the oral cavity because of the proximity to the salivary glands. It can be transient or permanent, depending on the radiation dose. Evidence shows that mean doses of less than 26 Gy to the parotid glands may prevent permanent xerostomia. Parotid and submandibular sparing requires three-dimensional approaches including intensity-modulated radiation therapy to reduce radiation exposure to normal tissue. Amifostine, a radioprotector given during radiation, has been shown to reduce acute grade 2 or greater xerostomia from 78% to 51% and chronic grade 2 or greater xerostomia from 57% to 34% ($P = .002$) without compromising tumor control [32].

Radiation mucositis usually occurs 2 to 4 weeks into treatment and abates 3 weeks to 2 months after the completion of radiation. Acute mucositis can be painful, and pain issues need to be addressed immediately to allow the patient to continue to eat. To minimize the chance of secondary infection, most radiation oncologists recommend baking soda mouthwash. Should secondary infections (most often thrush) occur, appropriate antibiotic treatment is initiated. Topical anesthetic mouthwashes provide pain relief for 10 to 30 minutes that may help with eating. Many patients require narcotic analgesia for adequate pain control. Mucositis often causes significant swelling, which may be managed by nonsteroidal anti-inflammatory agents or steroids. Usually, mucositis resolves 4 to 6 weeks after radiation is completed, but occasionally it can last for several months, necessitating close surveillance.

It is now a common practice to place a gastrostomy feeding tube before the start of chemoradiation therapy for food supplementation or replacement. This precaution often prevents excessive weight loss and dehydration and ultimately prevents an unwanted treatment interruption. Nutritional and volume status need to be watched closely through treatment.

Finally, skin reactions need to be addressed in most head and neck patients receiving chemoradiation therapy. Skin moisturizers, antibiotic cream, and topical anesthetics are usually used to help patients who have severe skin reactions.

Dental care

It is critical that, before starting radiation, all patients are evaluated by a dentist who has experience in managing head and neck cancer patients. Dental extraction may be required, and daily fluoride therapy often is initiated during and after radiation therapy to reduce the risk of future tooth decay and the development of osteoradionecrosis.

Treatment of oral cavity cancer

Treatment of early-stage disease

Brachytherapy

In patients who have small oral cavity lesions (T1/T2 N0), surgical resection is considered the standard of care. For patients who have a true T1/T2 N0 lesion, adjuvant radiation therapy is not indicated when adequate surgical margins are achieved and the patient has no risk factors for locoregional recurrence such as perineural invasion/lymphovascular invasion. Patients with early-stage disease who are poor surgical candidates can be treated with interstitial brachytherapy alone. The most commonly used radiation source is Ir[192]. Lefebvre and colleagues [9] reported the local control rates from a large series with 579 patients presenting with early oral cancer treated at Centre Oscar Lambret. Of these patients, 429 were treated locally by brachytherapy; local control was achieved in 82% of the cases. Treatment-related complications occurred in 19% of the cases. Other series with small patient numbers also reported local control rates of 80% to 90% in the patients who had early-stage oral cavity cancer treated with brachytherapy [10,11].

In patients who have early-stage disease treated with surgical resection with close or positive margins, adjuvant interstitial brachytherapy can result in local control and overall survival rates similar to those in patients who have completely resected tumors. Lapeyre and colleagues [11] reported on 82 patients who had positive or close margins after surgical resection who received postoperative brachytherapy. Forty-six patients had combined external beam radiotherapy and brachytherapy boost. Thirty-six patients had brachytherapy alone with a mean dose of 60 Gy. Brachytherapy was performed with interstitial low-dose-rate Ir[192]. The local control rate at 5 years was 88% for patients who had T1/T2 N0 tumors treated with brachytherapy alone for close or positive surgical margins.

External beam radiation with brachytherapy

For more advanced disease, the disadvantage of brachytherapy alone is the inadequate coverage for regional sites at high risk for tumor dissemination. Clinical T1/T2 N0 oral cavity cancer is associated with an occult lymph node metastasis rate of about 25%. In a report by Brugere and colleagues [12] of 826 patients who had squamous cell carcinoma of the oral cavity, all clinically N0, the primary tumor was treated by resection or brachytherapy. All patients underwent cervical dissection adapted to the site of the tumor. Two hundred patients were found to have lymph node metastasis, for an occult lymph node metastasis rate of 24%.

Depending on risk factors, a patient who has early-stage oral cavity cancer may require surgical resection followed by external beam radiation alone to the areas at high risk for lymphatic spread or with brachytherapy as a boost to the primary tumor site. Most series reported a mixed patient population with early-stage oral cavity cancer treated with surgery, brachytherapy, external beam radiation, or a combination of these modalities. In a series of 1344 cases of carcinoma of the oral cavity and oropharynx, brachytherapy was performed with Ir[192], either alone or in combination with external beam irradiation or surgery for the treatment of the primary tumor. For the oral cavity, 565 cases of mobile tongue were studied. The 5-year local control and overall survival rates, respectively, were 92% and 70% for T1 disease and 62% and 42% for T2 disease [14]. Similar reports show excellent local control in this patient population treated with combined modalities [13,14].

In centers without brachytherapy equipment or expertise, external beam radiation therapy alone can be used in early-stage patients who have high risk factors (close or positive margins, perineural/lymphovascular invasion, or lymph node metastasis) after surgical resection.

Treatment of locally advanced disease

Many patients present with locally advanced disease, defined as T3/T4 lesions or spread to the regional lymph nodes with or without extracapsular extension. Most of the recent trials addressing the role of radiotherapy in head and neck cancer involve patients who have locally advanced disease. The remainder of this article discusses the issues regarding radiotherapy in locally advanced squamous cell carcinoma of the oral cavity. There are no prospective studies designed specifically for patients who have oral cavity cancer. Most of the articles referenced in this review pertain to head and neck cancer in general, but all articles referenced include carcinomas of the oral cavity.

Definitive chemoradiation therapy

During the past decade, many trials have evaluated the role of chemotherapy in combination with radiation in the definitive or adjuvant setting for patients who have locally advanced head and neck cancer. Many of these trials included patients with cancers of the oral cavity, and inferences can be made from these trials regarding the management of oral cavity carcinoma. Following are summaries of the major trials that have included carcinoma of the oral cavity.

In 2000, Pignon [15] published a landmark meta-analysis of 63 trials looking at the value of chemotherapy when added to definitive radiotherapy for head and neck cancer. The meta-analysis included trials that compared radiation alone with radiation in conjunction with neoadjuvant, concurrent, or adjuvant chemotherapy; trials comparing different schedules of chemotherapy and radiation; and larynx-preservation trials incorporating chemotherapy. Chemotherapy offered an absolute overall survival benefit of 4% at both 2 years (54% versus 50%) and 5 years (36% versus 32%; $P < .0001$). Concurrent chemotherapy accounted for the majority of the benefit, with an absolute survival benefit of 7% at 2 years and of 8% at 5 years ($P < .0001$). Neither neoadjuvant nor adjuvant chemotherapy provided a statistically significant survival benefit. In subgroup analysis, the survival benefit of chemotherapy was observed for patients who had advanced carcinomas of the oral cavity. Based on laboratory data, investigators postulate that the benefit of concurrent chemotherapy stems from the radiosensitizing effects of cisplatin-based chemotherapy, which translates into improved local control and ultimately into improved overall survival. Although this study was a meta-analysis, it made a convincing argument for concurrent chemoradiation therapy in the treatment of locally advanced carcinoma of the head and neck.

To further define the benefit of concurrent chemoradiotherapy, Jeremic [1] published a three-arm randomized trial involving 159 patients who had locally advanced squamous cell carcinoma of the head and neck. Patients were randomly assigned to definitive radiotherapy alone to 70 Gy or to the same radiotherapy with either daily cisplatin (6 mg/m^2) or carboplatin (25 mg/m^2) given on days that the patients were receiving radiation. Compared with the radiation-only arm, both chemoradiation arms showed statistically significant benefits in terms of 5-year local recurrence-free survival (51% and 48% respectively, versus 27%) and 5-year overall survival (32% and 29% respectively, versus 15%). The median survival time was 30 months for the carboplatin arm, 32 months for the cisplatin arm, and only 16 months for the radiotherapy-alone arm ($P = .019$; $P = .011$). There was no difference between the three groups in the rate of distant metastases or nodal recurrences. Both chemoradiation groups had higher rates of hematologic toxicity than the radiation-only group. There were no significant differences between the carboplatin and cisplatin arms in terms of outcomes or toxicities.

More recent trials have established chemoradiation as the standard of care for patients who have locally advanced head and neck cancer and who are interested in organ preservation or are deemed inoperable. In 2003, Adelstein [2] reported a similar three-arm randomized trial in patients who had locally advanced squamous cell carcinoma of the head and neck, comparing standard radiation alone (70 Gy) with two schedules of concurrent chemoradiation. One arm received concurrent cisplatin (100 mg/m^2) on days 1, 22, 43 of radiation to 70 Gy. The other arm received multiagent chemotherapy with three courses of cisplatin (75 mg/m^2) and 5-fluorouracil (5-FU) (1000 mg/m^2) with a split course of radiation with of a break after 30 Gy and then continuing radiation to 60 to 70 Gy. The 3-year overall survival was significantly worse in the radiation therapy–only arm (23%) than in the cisplatin/radiation therapy arm (37%; $P = 0.014$). Once again, the survival benefit came at a cost of significant acute toxicity in the chemoradiation arms. The survival benefit was not seen in the cisplatin/5-FU/split-course radiation therapy arm, probably because of tumor cell–accelerated repopulation during the break in radiation treatment. This trial further supports the benefit of chemotherapy delivered concurrently with radiation.

To evaluate the response and toxicity of various chemoradiotherapeutic regimens, the Radiation Therapy Oncology Group (RTOG) initiated a randomized phase II trial comparing three concurrent chemotherapy regimens in patients who had locally advanced carcinoma of the oral cavity, oropharynx, and hypopharynx [16]. Radiation was 70 Gy using standard 2-Gy fractions, 5 d/wk, in all treatment arms. Patients in arm 1 received cisplatin (10 mg/m^2/d) and 5-FU (400 mg/m^2 continuous infusion) for the last 10 days of radiation. Patients in arm 2 received hydroxyurea (1 g every 12 hours) and 5-FU (800 mg/m^2 every day of radiation). Patients in arm 3 received paclitaxel (30 mg/m^2) and cisplatin (20 mg/m^2) weekly. Patients in arms 1 and 3 received radiation in 7 consecutive weeks; patients in arm 2 had alternating weeks of radiation over 13 weeks. This trial showed acceptable toxicities in all the arms, indicating feasibility of all regimens. Although this trial was not designed to address efficacy, the estimated 2-year overall survival rates were similar in all treatment arms (cisplatin/5-FU: 57.4%; hydroxyurea/ 5-FU: 69.4%; paclitaxel/cisplatin: 66.6%). Most cooperative group studies incorporate a cisplatin-based regimen; however, as this study demonstrates, patients who may not tolerate cisplatin clearly have alternative chemotherapy options. Overall, these studies show that, in patients who have locally advanced carcinoma of the head and neck, concurrent chemoradiation therapy offers a significant survival benefit over radiation alone at the expense of higher acute toxicities.

Altered fractionation

The use of altered fractionation radiation, defined as the delivery of more than one fraction of radiation daily, has been investigated in the management of head and neck cancer during the past decade. The rationale for altered fractionation is that a higher radiation dose can be delivered in a shorter period of time, and normal tissue can recover from radiation damage to a certain degree during the interfraction interval. Thus, in theory, altered fractionation should improve tumor control without increasing long-term side effects. There are many ways to alter conventional fractionation consisting of 1.8- to 2-Gy daily fractions. Hyperfractionation refers to the use of smaller doses per fraction, usually given twice daily. Accelerated fractionation refers to a shortened overall treatment duration without a decrease in the total dose, usually done by increasing the dose given per fraction. Concomitant boost fractionation is a combination of hyperfractionation and accelerated fractionation, taking advantage of the radiobiologic concept of accelerated repopulation of surviving tumor cells after 3 to 4 weeks of radiation. Typically, concomitant boost fractionation consists of conventional fractionation to a large field for the first 3.5 weeks followed by 2.5 weeks of twice-daily treatments given at least 6 hours apart, one to the initial large field and one to a smaller boost field.

RTOG 9003 explored altered fractionation by randomly assigning 1113 patients who had locally advanced squamous cell carcinoma of the head and neck to one of four fractionation schemes [5]:

1. Conventional standard fractionation (70 Gy in daily 2-Gy fractions)
2. Hyperfractionation (81.6 Gy in twice-daily 1.2-Gy fractions)
3. Concomitant boost (72 Gy consisting of daily 1.8-Gy fractions with a second daily fraction of 1.5 Gy delivered to a smaller field on the last 12 days of therapy)
4. Accelerated fractionation delivered in a split-course fashion (67.2 Gy in twice-daily 1.6-Gy fractions with a 2-week rest after 38.4 Gy)

At 23 months, both hyperfractionation and concomitant boost fractionation showed improved local control compared with standard fractionation

($P = .045$ and .050, respectively). Split-course fractionation, however, showed local control equivalent to standard fractionation, a result thought to be caused by accelerated repopulation of the tumor cells during the treatment break. There was a trend toward improved disease-free survival with concomitant boost and hyperfractionation compared with standard fractionation, but there was no overall survival difference between the four arms. Grade 3 and higher acute toxicities were significantly higher in all three experimental arms; however, late toxicities (defined as toxicities $>$ 6 months after radiation) were similar among all treatment arms. Overall, this trial showed that, in patients who have locally advanced head and neck cancer, hyperfractionation and concomitant boost fractionation result in improved local control compared with conventional fractionation, at the cost of increased acute toxicities.

Hyperfractionated radiation with chemotherapy

With many trials showing a survival benefit with concurrent chemotherapy, radiation oncology investigators have explored the tolerability and efficacy of combining concurrent chemotherapy with altered fractionation radiation.

Investigators at Duke University randomly assigned 122 patients with locally advanced head and neck cancer to hyperfractionated radiation alone (75 Gy in twice-daily 1.25-Gy fractions) or to hyperfractionated radiation plus chemotherapy (70 Gy in twice-daily fractions with 5-FU, 600 mg/m^2/d, and cisplatin, 12 mg/m^2/d, during weeks 1 and 6, and with two cycles of chemotherapy following radiation) [6]. Chemotherapy significantly improved 3-year locoregional control (70% versus 44%; $P = .01$) and trended toward improving 3-year relapse-free survival (61% versus 41%; $P = .08$) and overall survival (55% versus 34%; $P = .07$). Need for a feeding tube was higher in patients receiving chemotherapy, and one patient in the chemotherapy group died of sepsis. Other acute and long-term side effects, including incidence of mucositis, were similar in the two arms. There seemed to be a slight imbalance in the arm receiving hyperfractionated radiation alone, with a greater cohort of patients presenting with N2/3 disease (61% versus 44%), but even after adjustment for nodal status, there was an improved local control rate with concurrent chemotherapy. Overall, this trial showed that concurrent chemotherapy improved local control, at the expense of increased reliance on feeding tubes and higher risk of myclosuppression.

A more recent study from Yugoslavia showed an overall survival benefit when chemotherapy was added to hyperfractionated radiotherapy [7]. This trial randomly assigned 130 patients who had stage III/IV squamous cell carcinoma of the head and neck to hyperfractionated radiation alone (77 Gy in twice-daily 1.1-Gy fractions) or to hyperfractionated radiation with concomitant chemotherapy (same radiation with daily cisplatin, 6 mg/m^2). Concurrent chemotherapy significantly improved all 5-year endpoints, including overall survival (46% versus 25%), progression-free survival (46%

versus 25%), locoregional progression–free survival (50% versus 36%), and distant metastasis–free survival (86% versus 57%). Acute hematologic toxicities again were higher in the chemotherapy arm, as expected. Other acute toxicities and all late toxicities were similar in the two arms.

The RTOG initiated a phase II trial to evaluate the response and toxicity of using concomitant boost radiation with concurrent cisplatin-based chemotherapy. Concomitant boost offers the advantage of an overall shorter treatment time than hyperfractionated radiation, which requires twice-daily therapy at the outset. Cisplatin (100 mg/m^2) was administered on days 1 and 22 of radiation with concomitant boost radiotherapy, consisting of treating a large field to 54 Gy in 1.8-Gy daily fractions, with a twice-daily boost of 1.5 Gy/d to the gross disease and involved lymph nodes for the last 12 treatments. The total dose to the high-risk areas was 72 Gy [17]. Estimated 2-year overall survival was 71.6%, and 2-year locoregional control was 65.3%. Toxicities were similar to those seen in historical traditional chemoradiation trials. This experience led the RTOG to conduct a randomized phase III trial, RTOG 0129, comparing traditional once-daily radiation therapy with concurrent chemotherapy to concomitant boost radiation with concurrent chemotherapy. This trial recently achieved its accrual goals, and the results will be available in the next several years.

Postoperative chemoradiation therapy

In patients who have high-risk features, recurrence after surgery for head and neck cancer remains a problem. When evidence of perineural invasion is documented, recurrence rates as high as 80% have been reported in apparently completely resected T1/T2 tumors [18]. Indications for postoperative radiation include T3/T4 lesions, close or positive surgical margins, perineural invasion, lymphovascular invasion, multiple positive lymph nodes, or extracapsular extension. The presence of one or more of these risk factors qualifies a patient for postoperative radiation. Because of the extensive data supporting the addition of chemotherapy to radiation in the definitive setting, two trials have recently been published regarding the role of adding chemotherapy to radiation in the postoperative setting.

RTOG 9501 randomly assigned 459 patients who had squamous cell carcinoma of the head and neck who had undergone macroscopic resection of the tumor and had high-risk features (multiple positive lymph nodes, extracapsular extension, positive margins) to adjuvant radiation (60–66 Gy in once-daily 2-Gy fractions) or adjuvant concurrent chemoradiation (same radiation with concurrent cisplatin, 100 mg/m^2, on days 1, 22, and 43) [3]. With a median follow-up of 46 months, concurrent chemoradiation significantly improved 2-year local and regional control (82% versus 72%; $P = .01$) and disease-free survival ($P = .04$), but overall survival was not significantly different ($P = .19$). Chemotherapy resulted in significantly increased grade 3 or greater acute toxicities, 77% versus 34% (Fig. 1), but late toxicities were similar.

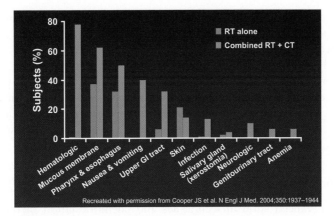

Fig. 1. The effects of combined modality therapy result in a significant increase in acute toxicity in patients treated in the postoperative setting in RTOG 95-01. CT, chemotherapy; GI, gastrointestinal; RT, radiotherapy.

The European Organization for Research and Treatment of Cancer (EORTC) conducted a similar trial, EORTC 22931, enrolling 334 patients who had high risk factors after resection of squamous cell carcinoma of the head and neck comparing radiation (66 Gy) versus a similar radiation dose and concurrent cisplatin (100 mg/m^2) on days 1, 22, and 43 [4]. In contrast to RTOG 9501, this study did show a significant 5-year overall survival benefit to concurrent cisplatin chemotherapy in the postoperative setting (53% versus 40%; $P = .02$). Of note were the differences in the definitions of high-risk disease (Fig. 2). Functional mucosal adverse effects and myelosuppression were higher in the combined treatment arm, but the cumulative incidence of late complications was similar in the two groups. A recent analysis and comparison of the two trials indicated that chemoradiation was beneficial in patients who have extracapsular extension or microscopically

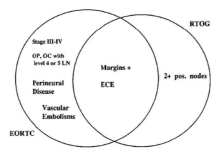

Fig. 2. Eligibility criteria for EORTC 22931 and RTOG 9501. ECE, extracapsular extension; LN, lymph nodes; OC, oral cavity; OP, oropharynx. (*From* Bernier J, Cooper JS, Pajak TF, et al. Defining risk levels in locally advanced head and neck cancers: a comparative analysis of concurrent postoperative radiation plus chemotherapy trials of the EORTC (#22931) and RTOG (#9501). Head Neck 2005;27:843–50; with permission.)

positive margins. Patients who have the risk factor of two or more positive lymph nodes, without extracapsular extension, did not experience a survival benefit from chemoradiation [19].

Overall, in postoperative patients who have high risk factors, chemoradiation provides a disease-free survival benefit and probably an overall survival benefit. This benefit comes at the cost of increased acute side effects. Therefore, it is important that a multidisciplinary approach be taken with high-risk patients in an effort to individualize treatment recommendations based on disease extent, performance status, and comorbidities.

Future directions

With advanced surgical techniques and chemoradiation therapy, treatment outcome in locally advanced head and neck cancer as a whole has improved. Unfortunately, locally advanced head and neck cancer is still associated with unacceptably high locoregional recurrence rates, and more than 50% of the patients die from tumor persistence, recurrence, or progression. Additionally, severe complications accompany aggressive treatment. Understanding tumorigenesis, tumor progression, and metastasis on a molecular level will ultimately refine the treatment of head and neck cancer, increasing treatment effectiveness and decreasing treatment-related toxicities.

McGregor and colleagues [20] reported that half of oral dysplasia cultures are immortal, and this immortality is associated with loss of expression of retinoic acid receptor-beta and the cell cycle inhibitor p16, p53 mutations, and increased levels of telomerase/human telomerase reverse transcriptase mRNA [20]. Emerging data also indicate that EGFR and its signal transduction pathway may play an important role in head and neck cancer. Expression of EGFR is increased in head and neck tumor cells and even in the tumor-adjacent epithelium. Van Oijen and colleagues [21] found that the closer the head and neck cancer cells are to the epithelium, the higher is the expression of the EGFR. EGFR expression itself has been proven to be an independent prognostic factor in local control and overall survival in patients who have locally advanced head and neck cancer [22]. Overexpression of EGFR correlated significantly with lower tumor grade and poor prognosis [23]. EGFR overexpression has also been shown to be statistically associated with T stage, N stage, overall TMN stage, primary tumor depth, and lymph node extracapsular spread [24]. The increased capacity for EGF binding may also play an important role in the tumorigenesis of head and neck cancer [25].

Of relevance to the radiation oncologist is that radiation has been observed to activate EGFR signaling [26] which may contribute to the rapid repopulation seen in surviving cancer clonogens. The rationale for blocking EGFR signaling lies in the preclinical data that demonstrated the correlation of EGFR expression and radiation resistance in vivo [27,28]. Fig. 3 demonstrates the interaction of EGFR inhibitors with the cell-signaling

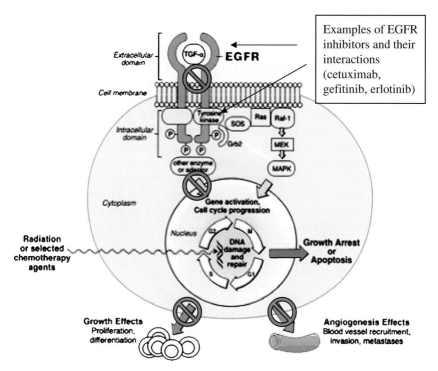

Fig. 3. EGFR blockade results in inhibition of downstream signaling within the cancer cell that results in reduced proliferation, angiogenesis, invasion, and an increase in apoptosis. TGF-α, transforming growth factor alpha.

pathways. Overexpression of EGFR is associated with increased malignant potential and correlates with poor clinical outcome in head and neck cancer [29]. Therefore, inhibition of the EGFR pathway provides an ideal target for molecular therapy. In oral cavity cancers, EGFR blockade arrests the growth of oral cancer in vitro and reduces its proliferation in experimental xenograft animal models [30].

These concepts have been translated successfully to the clinic. Recent data from a phase III trial presented at the 2004 annual meeting of the American Society of Clinical Oncology showed a significant improvement in overall survival with the addition of a humanized anti-EGFR monoclonal antibody, cetuximab, to radiation therapy in patients with advanced head and neck cancer [8]. There seemed to be no significant increase in mucositis and only a modest increase in skin toxicity with the addition of cetuximab weekly over radiation alone, far less than typically observed with concurrent chemoradiation.

Small molecules such as gefitinib and erlotinib, which block the EGFR signal transduction pathway, are in the early clinical trials of head and neck cancer treatment. Preliminary results showed that gefitinib is well tolerated by patients who have locally advanced head and neck cancer and who are receiving radiation therapy or concurrent chemoradiation therapy [31]. An ongoing multicenter, double-blinded, randomized phase II study is comparing gefitinib with placebo in patients who have head and neck cancer and who are receiving chemoradiation therapy.

The use of targeted agents such as gefitinib and erlotinib, which have toxicity profiles different from those of conventional chemotherapy agents, would decrease hematologic toxicity and perhaps allow a more effective delivery of radiation therapy (eg, without treatment breaks). Under investigation is the addition of EGFR inhibitors to chemoradiation. With the survival benefit seen with cetuximab and radiation therapy, this strategy offers an exciting alternative to conventional approaches. Patient selection will be critical in future trial design to better predict which patients will respond best to a chemoradiation approach or to an approach using agents targeting growth signaling, such as the EGFR pathway.

Summary

Oral cavity cancer presents a therapeutic challenge to the treating surgeons, radiation oncologists, and medical oncologists. In early-stage disease, surgery or radiation alone often achieves excellent local control. Patients who have risk factors for recurrence after surgery should undergo adjuvant radiotherapy or chemoradiotherapy. In locally advanced disease, recurrence rates and deaths caused by disease progression continue to be unacceptably high. During the past decade, multiple randomized studies have shown a benefit in the addition of chemotherapy to radiation in the definitive or postoperative setting. Also, hyperfractionated and concomitant boost radiotherapy has shown superior results when compared with conventional once-daily radiotherapy. The addition of chemotherapy to hyperfractionated or concomitant boost radiotherapy also seems to improve outcomes at the cost of increased toxicities. In addition to traditional therapeutic modalities, new targeted agents seem promising to improve outcomes and possibly allow use of decreased doses of chemotherapy or radiotherapy, thus decreasing the toxicity of treatment. Overall, the management of cancer of the oral cavity is evolving rapidly, and a multidisciplinary approach to the patient who has oral cavity cancer is important to ensure the highest quality of patient care.

References

[1] Jeremic B, Shibamoto Y, Stanisavljevic B, et al. Radiation therapy alone or with concurrent low-dose daily either cisplatin or carboplatin in locally advanced unresectable squamous cell carcinoma of the head and neck: a prospective randomized trial. Radiother Oncol 1997;43: 29–37.
[2] Adelstein DJ, Adams GL, Wagner H, et al. An intergroup phase III comparison of standard radiation therapy and two schedules of concurrent chemoradiotherapy in patients with unresectable squamous cell head and neck cancer. J Clin Oncol 2003;21(1):92–8.

[3] Cooper JS, Pajak TF, Forastiere AA, et al. Postoperative concurrent radiotherapy and chemotherapy for high-risk squamous-cell carcinoma of the head and neck. N Engl J Med 2004; 350(19):1937–44.

[4] Bernier J, Domenge C, Ozsahin M, et al. Postoperative irradiation with or without concomitant chemotherapy for locally advanced head and neck cancer. N Engl J Med 2004;350(19): 1945–52.

[5] Fu KK, Pajak TF, Trotti A, et al. A Radiation Therapy Oncology Group phase III randomized study to compare hyperfractionation and two variants of accelerated fractionation to standard fractionation radiotherapy for head and neck squamous cell carcinomas: first report of RTOG 9003. Int J Radiat Oncol Biol Phys 2000;48(1):7–16.

[6] Brizel DM, Albers ME, Fisher SR, et al. Hyperfractionated irradiation with or without concurrent chemotherapy for locally advanced head and neck cancer. N Engl J Med 1998; 338(25):1798–804.

[7] Jeremic B, Shibamoto Y, Milicic B, et al. hyperfractionated radiation therapy with or without concurrent low-dose daily cisplatin in locally advanced squamous cell carcinoma of the head and neck: a prospective randomized trial. J Clin Oncol 2000;18(7):1458–64.

[8] Bonner JA, Giralt J, Harari PM, et al. Cetuximab prolongs survival in patients with locoregionally advanced squamous cell carcinoma of head and neck: a phase III study of high dose radiation therapy with or without cetuximab. J Clin Oncol 2004;22(14S):5507.

[9] Lefebvre JL, Coche-Dequeant B, Buisset E, et al. Management of early oral cavity cancer. Experience of Centre Oscar Lambret. Eur J Cancer B Oral Oncol 1994;30B(3):216–20.

[10] Wadsley JC, Patel M, Tomlins CD, et al. Iridium-192 implantation for T1 and T2a carcinoma of the tongue and floor of mouth: retrospective study of the results of treatment at the Royal Berkshire Hospital. Br J Radiol 2003;76(906):414–7.

[11] Lapeyre M, Bollet MA, Racadot S, et al. Postoperative brachytherapy alone and combined postoperative radiotherapy and brachytherapy boost for squamous cell carcinoma of the oral cavity, with positive or close margins. Head Neck 2004;26(3):216–23.

[12] Brugere JM, Mosseri VF, Mamelle G, et al. Nodal failures in patients with N0 N+ oral squamous cell carcinoma without capsular rupture. Head Neck 1996;18(2):133–7.

[13] Grabenbauer GG, Rodel C, Brunner T, et al. Interstitial brachytherapy with Ir-192 low-dose-rate in the treatment of primary and recurrent cancer of the oral cavity and oropharynx. Review of 318 patients treated between 1985 and 1997. Strahlenther Onkol 2001;177(7): 338–44.

[14] Rudoltz MS, Perkins RS, Luthmann RW, et al. High-dose-rate brachytherapy for primary carcinomas of the oral cavity and oropharynx. Laryngoscope 1999;109(12):1967–73.

[15] Pignon JP, Bourhis J, Domenge C, et al. Chemotherapy added to locoregional treatment for head and neck squamous-cell carcinoma: three meta-analyses of updated individual data. Lancet 2000;355:949–55.

[16] Garden AS, Harris J, Vokes EE, et al. Preliminary results of Radiation Therapy Oncology Group 97–03: a randomized phase II trial of concurrent radiation and chemotherapy for advanced squamous cell carcinomas of the head and neck. J Clin Oncol 2004;22(14): 2856–64.

[17] Ang KK, Harris J, Garden AS, et al. Concomitant boost radiation plus concurrent cisplatin for advanced head and neck carcinomas: Radiation Therapy Oncology Group phase II trial 99–14. J Clin Oncol 2005;23(13):3008–15.

[18] O'Brien C, Lahr C, Soong S, et al. Surgical treatment of early-stage carcinoma of the oral tongue: would adjuvant treatment be beneficial? Head Neck Surg 1986;8:401–8.

[19] Bernier J, Cooper JS, Pajak TF, et al. Defining risk levels in locally advanced head and neck cancers: a comparative analysis of concurrent postoperative radiation plus chemotherapy trials of the EORTC (#22931) and RTOG (#9501). Head Neck 2005;27:843–50.

[20] McGregor F, Muntoni A, Fleming J, et al. Molecular changes associated with oral dysplasia progression and acquisition of immortality: potential for its reversal by 5-azacytidine. Cancer Res 2002;62(16):4757–66.

[21] van Oijen MG, Rijksen G, ten Broek FW, et al. Increased expression of epidermal growth factor receptor in normal epithelium adjacent to head and neck carcinomas independent of tobacco and alcohol abuse. Oral Dis 1998;4(1):4–8.

[22] Ang KK, Berkey BA, Tu X, et al. Impact of epidermal growth factor receptor expression on survival and pattern of relapse in patients with advanced head and neck carcinoma. Cancer Res 2002;62:7350–6.

[23] Bankfalvi A, Krassort M, Vegh A, et al. Deranged expression of the E-cadherin/beta-catenin complex and the epidermal growth factor receptor in the clinical evolution and progression of oral squamous cell carcinomas. J Oral Pathol Med 2002;31(8):450–7.

[24] Chen IH, Chang JT, Liao CT, et al. Prognostic significance of EGFR and Her-2 in oral cavity cancer in betel quid prevalent area cancer prognosis. Br J Cancer 2003;89(4):681–6.

[25] Rikimaru K, Tadokoro K, Yamamoto T, et al. Gene amplification and overexpression of epidermal growth factor receptor in squamous cell carcinoma of the head and neck. Head Neck 1992;14(1):8–13.

[26] Schmit-Ullrich RK, Mikkelsen RB, Dent P, et al. Radiation-induced proliferation of the human A431 squamous carcinoma cells is dependent on EGFR tyrosine phosphorylation. Oncogene 1997;15:1191–7.

[27] Akimoto T, Hunter NR, Buchmiller L, et al. Inverse relationship between epidermal growth factor receptor expression and radiocurability of murine carcinomas. Clin Cancer Res 1999; 5(10):2884–90.

[28] Huang SM, Bock JM, Harari PM. Epidermal growth factor receptor blockade with C225 modulates proliferation, apoptosis, and radiosensitivity in squamous cell carcinomas of the head and neck. Cancer Res 1999;59(8):1935–40.

[29] Ang KK, Berkey BA, Tu X, et al. Impact of epidermal growth factor receptor expression on survival and pattern of relapse in patients with advanced head and neck carcinoma. Cancer Res 2002;62:7350–6.

[30] Myers JN, Holsinger FC, Bekele BN, et al. Targeted molecular therapy for oral cancer with epidermal growth factor receptor blockade: a preliminary report. Arch Otolaryngol Head Neck Surg 2002;128(8):875–9.

[31] Raben D, Chen C, Eckhardt GS, et al. Maturing toxicity and outcome of a phase I trial of concurrent, daily gefitinib and radiation or chemoradiation for patients with locally advanced squamous cell carcinoma of the head and neck (LASCCHN). Int J Radiat Oncol Biol Phys 2005;63(2):S370–1.

[32] Brizel DM, Wasserman TH, Henke M, et al. Phase II randomized trial of amifostine as a radioprotector in head and neck cancer. J Clin Oncol 2000;18(19):3339–45.

ELSEVIER
SAUNDERS

Otolaryngol Clin N Am
39 (2006) 381–396

OTOLARYNGOLOGIC
CLINICS
OF NORTH AMERICA

Future Directions in the Treatment of Oral Cancer

Wounjhang Park, PhD[a,b], Jonathan M. Owens, MD[c,*]

[a]Department of Electrical & Computer Engineering, University of Colorado, UCB 425,
Boulder, CO 80309-0425, USA
[b]University of Colorado Cancer Center, 1645 North Ursula Street, Denver 80045, CO, USA
[c]Department of Otolaryngology-Head and Neck Surgery, University of Colorado
Health Sciences Center, 4300 East 9th Avenue, Box B-205, Denver, CO 80262, USA

Oral cavity cancer has an incidence of 29,000 cases annually in the United States, with 7900 deaths [1]. Despite significant efforts in early detection and treatment of oral cancer in the past several decades, little change in overall survival has been afforded these patients. Contemporary treatment options include surgical resection, chemotherapy, and radiation therapy. Typically, multimodality therapy is used for more advanced or difficult lesions.

Recent technologic advances offer promise for future diagnostic and therapeutic modalities for patients who have oral cancer. Nanotechnology refers to the use of nanomaterials, which are defined by their size and are characterized by their unique properties that often are drastically different from their bulk counterpart. This technology and the possibilities that it offers are explored. Similarly, the explosion in the therapeutic application of molecular genetics and molecular biology has led to the development of gene microarrays. These devices promise the development of truly personalized cancer treatment that is based on the expression of particular genes by each individual tumor.

New directions based on nanotechnology

Nanomaterial refers to a newly emerging class of materials whose sizes are on the order of 10^{-9} meter, or 1/100,000th of the width of a human hair. This size range represents clusters of atoms or molecules that neither

This work was supported in part by the University of Colorado Cancer Center.
* Corresponding author.
E-mail address: jonathan.owens@uschc.edu (J.M. Owens).

0030-6665/06/$ - see front matter © 2005 Elsevier Inc. All rights reserved.
doi:10.1016/j.otc.2005.11.009

behave as macroscopic bulk material nor exhibit the characteristics of individual atoms or molecules. The unique characteristics of nanomaterials promise abundant opportunities for new scientific discoveries and novel engineering schemes. Although this tremendous potential was recognized many decades ago [2], it was only recently that nanoscience and nanotechnology have become a major research field. This is due, in part, to the lack or immaturity of the means with which scientists can explore nanoscale materials and phenomena. During the past decade, there has been tremendous growth and advance in nanoscience and nanotechnology. Our understanding of the physical and chemical properties of nanomaterials has increased greatly and, based on such knowledge, nanodevices and nanosystems are being researched and developed actively. These exciting developments and the recognition of the potential economic impact resulted in greater investment in this field. For example, the U.S. government established a federal initiative on nanoscience and nanotechnology in 2001 [3]. Consequently, infrastructures for nanoscience and nanotechnology are expanding and maturing rapidly, and finally, many commercial applications that are based on nanotechnology are being introduced. A recent National Research Council report predicted that nanotechnology will have dramatic impacts on nearly every sector of our economy [4].

Nanomaterials are attractive mainly because they tend to exhibit strongly enhanced optical, electrical, or magnetic properties. Furthermore, these intrinsic, and thus, generally unalterable material properties become "tunable" by engineering the size and shape of the nanomaterial. Thus, nanomaterials make an ideal material platform to realize precisely tailored materials that exhibit prescribed properties. This article provides a review of the applications of nanomaterials on cancer research and treatment.

Semiconductor quantum dots for fluorescence imaging

Development of high-sensitivity, high-specificity probes is of considerable interest in molecular/cellular biology, molecular imaging, and medical diagnostics. For this purpose, organic dyes, often called "fluorophors," have been used widely. In this scheme, the fluorophors are bound to specific tissues or molecules; they emit characteristic fluorescence at various wavelengths when excited by an external light source. The sensitivity of this fluorescence imaging technique is high; in a microscopy set-up, it is possible to detect a single molecule.

The fluorophors also exhibit some serious drawbacks. They degrade quickly, and thus, the fluorescence fades rapidly. In addition, the choice of fluorescence wavelength is constrained by the limited range of required excitation wavelength. Fluorescence, in general, requires excitation by an energy light source, and therefore, one often needs a UV light source to excite visible fluorescence. The UV light is absorbed strongly by biologic tissues and has a strong tendency to excite background fluorescence that often deteriorates the image quality. The best spectral window for excitation and fluorescence generally is believed to be the near infrared (NIR) region between 600 and 900 nm. In this window, light can penetrate tissues with minimal absorption or scattering up to a depth of 10 cm. Shorter wavelengths are absorbed readily by hemoglobin and longer wavelengths are absorbed by water.

To overcome these deficiencies of conventional fluorophors, extensive research recently has been conducted on semiconductor quantum dots (QDs). Semiconductor QDs are extremely small particles of CdSe or ZnS whose sizes are in the range of 1 to 10 nm [5]. After bioconjugation, their hydrodynamic radii reach 10 to 20 nm, but the conjugated QDs generally do not suffer from serious binding kinetic problems. Semiconductor QDs exhibit much greater brightness and stability compared with the conventional fluorophors. In addition, the excitation band is broad, whereas their emission spectrum is narrow with a well-defined emission wavelength. The greatest advantage of QDs is that the emission spectrum can be tuned by changing the particle size and composition. This is the so-called "quantum size effect" in which photogenerated electron–hole pairs are bound strongly by the small size of the QD particle, and consequently, their energy is increased from the normal value of the bulk material. The smaller the particle sizes, the larger the energy of the electron–hole pair, which shifts the resultant fluorescence to a shorter wavelength. The achievable colors and fluorescence spectra are shown in Fig. 1 [6]. Thanks to this size tunability, there exists a large degree of engineering freedom to obtain tailored optical properties for specific applications.

CdSe is the most widely used material for QDs. To obtain a good size distribution, the synthesis process generally is performed in an organic solvent, such as trioctylphosphine oxide (TOPO), at an elevated temperature. Size is controlled primarily by the amount of the injected precursor materials and the time that the nanocrystals are left in the solution to grow. To obtain high-quality QDs for practical applications, proper surface treatment is critical. For reduction of surface recombination and an increase in luminescence

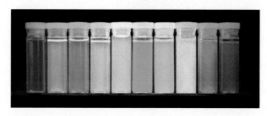

Fig. 1. Ten distinguishable emission colors of ZnS-capped CdSe QDs excited with a near-UV lamp. From left to right (blue to red), the emission maxima are located at 443, 473, 481, 500, 518, 543, 565, 587, 610, and 655 nm. (*From* Han M, Gao X, Su JZ, et al. Quantum-dot-tagged microbeads for multiplexed optical coding of biomolecules. Nat Biotechnol 2001;19:631; with permission.)

efficiency, thin ZnS coatings routinely are put on CdSe QDs. These CdSe-ZnS core-shell particles reach a quantum yield of approximately 80%. Another important requirement is to produce water-soluble QDs so that one can prepare aqueous QD colloidal solution. This is done by exchanging the hydrophobic TOPO surfactant molecules on the QD surface with bifunctional molecules that are hydrophilic on one end and bind to ZnS with the other end. A commonly used example is mercaptocarbonic acid, which has a thiol group to bind to ZnS and a carboxyl group for the hydrophilic surface [7]. The surface carboxyl group also is available for covalent bonding with various biomolecules, such as protein, peptides, and nucleic acids. A surface-treated QD particle is shown schematically in Fig. 2.

For biomedical applications, QD surfaces are modified further to target specific cells or molecules. QD–peptide conjugates have been used to target tumor vasculatures and homed to tumor vessels [8]. Antibody-conjugated QDs have been used for real-time imaging and tracking of molecules in living cells and demonstrated high sensitivity and resolution [9]. Most recently, QD probes were used for in vivo tumor targeting in passive and active modes [5]. In the passive targeting, QD probes are delivered and aggregated at tumor sites because of the enhanced permeability and retention effects. In the active mode, QD probes were conjugated with a prostate-specific membrane antigen (PSMA) monoclonal antibody to target PSMA preferentially, which is known as an attractive marker for prostate cancer. As shown in Fig. 3, successful targeting was demonstrated in both modes, but active targeting was faster and more efficient. After in vivo imaging, histologic and immunocytochemical examinations confirmed that the QD signals came from an underlying tumor. Similarly, QD probes could be conjugated to

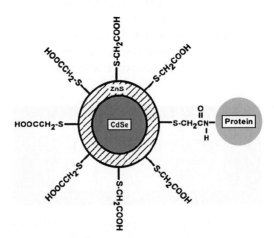

Fig. 2. A ZnS-capped CdSe QD coupled covalently to a protein by mercaptoacetic acid. (*From* Chan WCW, Nie S. Quantum dot bioconjugates for ultrasensitive nonisotopic detection. Science 1998;281:2016; with permission.)

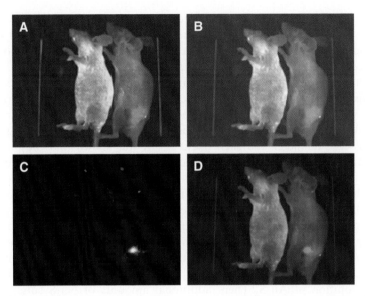

Fig. 3. Spectral imaging of conjugates of QD and prostate-specific membrane antigen antibody in live animals harboring C4-2 tumor xenografts. Orange-red fluorescence signals indicate a prostate tumor growing in a live mouse (*right*). Control studies using a healthy mouse (no tumor) and the same amount of QD injection showed no localized fluorescence signals (*left*). (*A*) Original image. (*B*) Unmixed autofluorescence image. (*C*) Unmixed QD image. (*D*) Superimposed image. (*From* Gao X, Cui Y, Levenson RM, et al. In vivo cancer targeting and imaging with semiconductor quantum dots. Nat Biotechnol 2004;22:969; with permission.)

monoclonal antibodies to oral cancer–specific antigens, such as epidermal growth factor receptor, to detect oral cancer cells specifically.

Metal nanoparticles and nanoshells

Metal nanoparticles have long been a subject of extensive research for their unique optical properties. The collective response of the electrons, known as the plasmon, gives rise to strong optical resonance and large and fast nonlinear optical polarizability. The optical properties are described well by the classic Mie theory [10] for the most part, and are the subject of much interest for their applications in, for example, optical filters [11], labeling in microscopy [12], and single-electron transistor [13]. In addition, the recently discovered enhanced Raman scattering has spurred extensive research activities [14].

The greatest usefulness of metal nanoparticles as an optical material arises from the fact that the strong plasmon resonance depends on particle geometry and the type of metal. Therefore, it is possible to control or "tune" the optical properties by the size and shape of the nanoparticles. For example, the well-known 520-nm plasmon resonance of gold nanoparticles shifts about 25 nm to longer wavelengths as the particle size is increased from 5 to

80 nm. The shift of plasmon resonance as a function of a solid metal particle's size tends to be small and, furthermore, controlling the size and shape of solid metal nanoparticles has been difficult, and good monodispersity has not been achieved for sizes greater than 100 nm [15].

Metal nanoshell, composed of a thin metal coating on a dielectric core, is a perfect alternative that provides much better control of size and shape and much wider tunability. The optical properties of metal nanoshells are described well by the Mie theory, and the plasmon resonance is a strong function of core diameter and shell thickness. It was shown that the plasmon resonance could be tuned from visible to beyond 10 μm in the far infrared [16].

Although the optical properties of metal nanoshells were known for decades [17], until recently the lack of reliable synthesis techniques prevented the experimental realization of high-quality nanoshells. In 1994, Zhou and colleagues [18] reported the formation of gold nanoshells on Au_2S cores using a two-step synthesis process. In this technique, controlled amounts of aqueous solutions of $HAuCl_4$ and Na_2S are mixed to obtain an unstable colloidal solution of Au_2S. Then, additional amounts of Na_2S solution are added to reduce Au ions on the surface of Au_2S nanoparticles. This process proceeds until all Au_2S core is reduced to Au, which produces gold nanoshells with various thicknesses. Consequently, the surface plasmon resonance shifted up to approximately 900 nm from the usual 520-nm peak of solid gold nanoparticles [19].

Although this is a convenient "one-pot" process for gold nanoshell synthesis, it is difficult to control the size and thickness of the nanoshells precisely. It is much more desirable to use dielectric cores with high monodispersity and then perform controlled growth of the nanoshell. This became possible by adopting the techniques of self-assembled monolayers and chemical modifications of dielectric and metallic surfaces. Oldenburg and colleagues [20] reported a synthesis technique that can produce gold nanoshells on silica core particles. Because the synthesis process for highly monodispersed silica nanoparticles is well established [21], using silica particles as the dielectric core provides precise control of the nanoshell's inner diameter. Graf and van Blaaderen [22] used a similar process and confirmed the formation of uniform and smooth gold nanoshells.

Following this strategy, we have synthesized gold nanoshells that exhibit strong tunable plasmon resonance. The process begins with the Stober synthesis of highly monodispersed silica spheres [21]. By controlling the temperature, precursor concentration, and pH precisely, we successfully synthesized silica spheres with diameters between 100 and 700 nm and monodispersity of less than 5%. Then, extremely small gold nanoparticles were synthesized by reducing gold with tetrakis(hydroxymethyl)phosphonium chloride, following the procedure that was similar to that first proposed by Duff and colleagues [23,24]. The preliminary results indicated that gold nanoparticles with diameters of approximately 2 nm were produced (Fig. 4a). Because of their small sizes, the optical extinction spectrum was featureless and the solution appeared yellow (see Fig. 4a).

To confirm this further, we intentionally increased the particle size by ripening at an elevated temperature. The nanoparticles then agglomerated and formed stable secondary structures. As the size became greater than 10 nm, the characteristic surface plasmon resonance of gold nanoparticle was observed at 520 nm, which turned the solution red. A further size increase caused a red shift of the plasmon peak. The colloidal solution turned blue and unstable (Fig. 4b).

The next step was to affix the small gold nanoparticles on the surface of silica spheres so that they would act as seeds for the subsequent shell growth process. To attract gold particles, the silica nanoparticles were treated with 3-aminopropyltrimethoxysilane. The silica surface is then terminated with amin group, which can bind small gold nanoparticles. The subsequent shell growth is performed by transferring the gold-attached silica spheres into an aqueous solution of $HAuCl_4$ and subsequently adding the reducing agent, $NH_2OH \cdot HCl$, dropwise. The seed gold nanoparticles attached on a silica surface start to grow through the reduction of the gold ion in the solution. Finally, a thin gold layer is formed on the silica core. During this process, the color of the solution changed from colorless to blue, green, or purple depending on the nanoshell size.

The nanoshells were characterized by scanning electron microscopy and optical spectroscopy. As shown in Fig. 5a and b, we obtained uniform and complete gold nanoshells without any holes or other nonuniformity. The extinction spectrum is another critical evidence for high quality of gold nanoshell. We dispersed the gold nanoshells in deionized water and maintained an adequate concentration ($\sim 10^8$ shells/mL). Fig. 5c shows

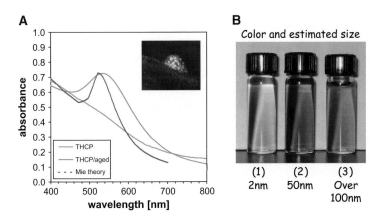

Fig. 4. (A) Experimental extinction spectra for small (~ 2 nm, purple) and large (~ 50 nm, red) gold nanoparticles. The theoretic spectrum calculated for 50-nm gold particles using the Mie theory (blue curve) also is shown. Inset: transmission electron microscope micrograph of gold nanoparticles with sizes of ~ 2 nm. (B) Color and estimated sizes of gold colloidal solution.

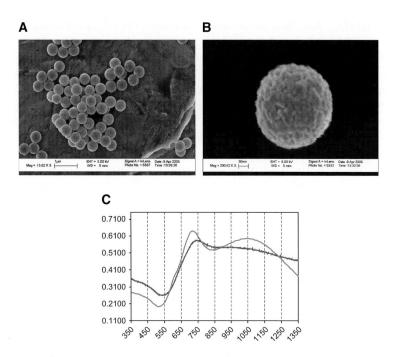

Fig. 5. Scanning electron microscope micrographs of gold nanoshells at low (*A*) and high (*B*) magnification. (*C*) Experimental (blue) and theoretic (red) extinction spectra of gold nanoshell with core diameter of 228 nm and shell thickness of 17 nm.

the extinction measurement result compared with the Mie scattering theory. The overall agreement between the theoretic and experimental spectra was good; however, the experimental spectrum was broadened because of the polydispersity, which we estimated to be 5%.

One of the most interesting characteristics of the nanoshells is that the plasmon resonance is tuned easily over the NIR "water window" (800–1300 nm), which represents the region of highest physiologic transmissivity. This makes these nanomaterials ideal for a variety of biomedical applications. An example is the nanoshell-embedded hydrogel that exhibits a dramatic optomechanical response [25]. A pure hydrogel does not absorb NIR light appreciably but, when nanoshells are embedded, it exhibits strong absorption that produces local heating. This results in a dramatic collapse, which is reversible and repeatable. This material system has a strong potential for laser-controlled drug delivery. Another example is nanoshell-mediated photothermal therapy. Nanoshells that absorb strongly in the water window can be used to respond selectively to the probing laser beam with minimal damage to the surrounding healthy tissues. Hirsch and colleagues [26] reported that gold nanoshells that were labeled with antibodies specific to oncoprotein were injected and bound to the target carcinoma cells.

Subsequent NIR illumination resulted in local heating because of strong absorption by the nanoshells and subsequent destruction of the tumor cells (Fig. 6).

Magnetic nanoparticles

MRI, which takes advantage of the magnetic properties of hydrogen in biologic tissues, is one of the most powerful and widely used imaging and diagnosis tools in medicine. Early in the development of MRI, it was believed that contrast agents would not be necessary; however, it has become clear that proper contrast agents can enhance the diagnostic value of MRI greatly [27].

The first generation of contrast agents is paramagnetic ions, usually Gd^{3+}, in various chelate forms. Gd^{3+} is preferred because it has seven unpaired 4f electrons, and therefore, it is strongly paramagnetic. The presence of Gd^{3+} ions primarily influences the T_1-relaxation process, which refers to the process of proton depolarization along the static magnetic field direction after the termination of transverse radiofrequency field pulse. In the close proximity of Gd^{3+} ions, the hydrogen atoms in water exhibit a significantly

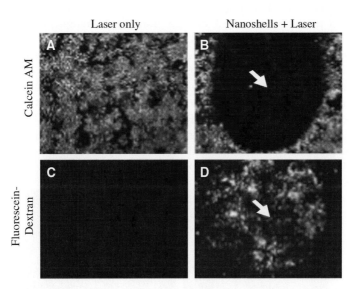

Fig. 6. Cells irradiated in the absence of nanoshells maintained viability, as depicted by calcein fluorescence (*A*), and membrane integrity, as indicated by lack of intracellular fluoroscein dextran uptake (*C*). Cells irradiated with nanoshells possess well-defined circular zones of cell death in the calcein AM study (*B*) and cellular uptake of fluoroscein dextran from increased membrane permeability (*D*). (*From* Hirsch LR, Stafford RJ, Bankson JA, et al. Nanoshell-mediated near-infrared thermal therapy of tumors under magnetic resonance guidance. Proc Natl Acad Sci USA 2003;100:13549; with permission.)

shortened T_1-relaxation process, which results in enhanced contrast in the T_1-weighted image.

Although T_1-weighted images can discriminate tissues with short T_1 (eg, fat) from those with long T_1 (eg, cerebrospinal fluid), tissues and fluids that often are associated with pathologies (eg, internal injuries and cancer lesions), tend to exhibit very long relaxation times for the T_2-decay process—the decay of transverse spin components upon termination of transverse radiofrequency magnetic field pulse. Therefore, T_2-weighted images are preferred for the diagnostics of cancer and internal injuries.

It was reported recently that magnetic nanoparticles are effective contrast enhancement agents for T_2-weighted images. The magnetic nanoparticles are 3- to 10-nm iron oxide particles that are coated with hydrophilic macromolecules, such as dextran and starch [28,29]. The macromolecules help to produce narrow size distribution by limiting the core particle growth and stabilize the nanoparticle colloid by providing steric repulsion. It also was found that the lethal dose for dextran–iron oxide complex is an order of magnitude larger than that of pristine iron oxide [30].

Often, these magnetic nanoparticles are called superparamagnetic because they exhibit magnetic moments that are much greater than those of conventional paramagnetic materials. This naturally leads to much greater relaxivity (ie, the capability to enhance the relaxation rate of protons) than Gd^{3+}-chelates. When the superparamagnetic nanoparticles are injected into target tissue, they create a strongly nonuniform magnetic field that induces dephasing of proton magnetic moment. This results in a significant reduction of T_2-relaxation time. Lee and colleagues [31] recently reported the synthesis of polylactide-co-glycolide (PLGA)-coated iron oxide nanoparticles using an emulsification–diffusion technique. By injecting the PLGA-coated magnetic nanoparticles into a rabbit, we showed a strong enhancement in the contrast of MRI images (Fig. 7).

Recently, the possibility of using superparamagnetic nanoparticles to induce hyperthermia or thermal ablation that is triggered by a magnetic field

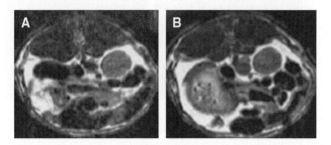

Fig. 7. MRI images (T_2) in the kidney of rabbit without (*A*) and with (*B*) PLGA-encapsulated iron oxide nanoparticles. (*From* Lee S-J, Jeong J-R, Shin S-C, et al. Nanoparticles of magnetic ferric oxides encapsulated with poly(D,L latide-co-glycolide) and their applications to magnetic resonance imaging contrast agent. J Magn Magn Mater 2004;272–276:2432.)

also has been investigated [32]. Because a magnetic field is not particularly transinduced for humans, it is considered one of the most ideal means to probe and to treat deep, scattered injuries or tumors. The superparamagnetic nanoparticles that exhibit strong absorption profiles can be used to produce local heating upon application of radiofrequency magnetic field without any significant influence or interference with the normal tissues. The current issues in the magnetic nanoparticle technology are better control of the synthesis process for highly monodispersed, strongly paramagnetic particles and the development of a surface conjugation process for specific targeting.

New directions in tumor diagnosis

Microarray/biostaging

The recent acceleration in genomic-based bioengineering products has included the development of the gene microarray. A gene microarray involves arranging a cDNA library of several hundred or several thousand gene sequence probes in a high-density two-dimensional array. mRNA is harvested from the tissue of interest and is reverse transcribed to double-stranded biotinylated DNA. This DNA is fragmented to create single-stranded target segments, which are exposed to the gene microarray, with complementary sequences of probe and target hybridizing to double-stranded product. Biotinylated secondary antibodies are applied, which is followed by fluorescent-labeled streptavidin staining of the hybridized products. Fluorescent scanning is used to quantify the staining of each site of the microarray, which quantifies the expression of the corresponding gene for each probe [33]. Alternatively, the reverse-transcribed DNA or the mRNA itself may be labeled with a fluorescent tag for detection [34].

Microarray technology allows the evaluation of the expression of thousands of genes by a given tissue in a single experiment. This enables the researcher to evaluate target genes in any given tissue with a "shotgun" approach. The relative expression of each gene, analyzed for each given tissue, contributes to a composite expression profile that can be compared with other tissue samples. The set of genes whose transcription differs between normal mucosa and malignant or premalignant samples may be used to create an index or genetic predictor for any new sample to be studied [34]. This sort of analysis has been performed with oral squamous cell cancers and normal mucosa. Three hundred and fourteen genes were expressed differentially in cancer tissue versus normal mucosa; the expression of 239 genes was upregulated and the expression of 75 genes was down-regulated in cancer specimens [35]. The investigators were able to use this profile to identify 23 new samples correctly as carcinoma or normal tissue in a subsequent report [34]. The greater statistical power of this method, compared with evaluating single biomarkers with immuno-histochemistry or polymerase chain reaction detection methods, is obvious.

Analysis of gene expression as determined by microarray analysis has been used to identify clusters of genes whose differential expression corre-lates with higher T-stage tumors [36], propensity of tumor for regional nodal metastasis [36–38], and predictive cause-specific survival [39].

The genes that were identified as being expressed significantly differentially by squamous cell carcinomas include those that are known to be associated with tumorigenesis as well as some genes that have not been implicated in tumor development or progression. Identification of these genes may direct further studies into the role of each one in the tumor process, and ultimately, may lead to future therapeutic development. Furthermore, identification of genes that portend more aggressive clinical behavior and regional metastasis of any given tumor may direct current therapy. For example, a patient who has clinically negative nodal disease, whose tumor is identified by microarray analysis to have increased potential for nodal metastasis, might be treated with elective neck dissection or irradiation, whereas one whose tumor does not possess such potential might be spared this adjuvant treatment.

Photodiagnosis

Oral mucosa undergoes an orderly progression in the development of in-vasive squamous cell carcinoma. Dysplasia is the earliest premalignant state, which may be followed by leukoplakia or erythroplakia. Progression to car-cinoma in situ and invasive squamous cell carcinoma may occur in any of these premalignant lesions. Obviously, early detection of small rests of inva-sive carcinoma in clinically suspicious lesions allows for treatment of these cancers at earlier stages, which would improve survival.

Various methods that incorporate fluorescence for tumor detection have been reported. Fluorescence spectroscopy of dysplastic mucosa in the hamster cheek pouch carcinogenesis model has been demonstrated. The ex-citation of this tissue with a 410-nm laser induces a fluorescence peak in the 630- to 640-nm range [40]. The fluorescence spectroscopy technique was confirmed by comparing the emission spectra of normal human oral mucosa and oral premalignant and malignant lesions following laser excitation at various frequencies [41,42].

Techniques that involve the application of free chromophore molecules to tissue have been in use for some time in photodynamic therapy, but these suffer from a lack of specificity. More modern techniques that are intended to alleviate this issue use a tumor-specific monoclonal antibody to which a fluorescent molecule is conjugated. Ideally, the probe binds only to tumor cells by virtue of expression of a specific target. Light of the appropriate wavelength for the given chromophore is applied to the tissue and fluores-cence is noted from the tumor. The first report of this technique in human cancer detection involved fluoresceinated antibodies to carcinoembryonic antigen for the detection of colorectal cancer [43]. Techniques that incorporated monoclonal antibodies that target the epidermal growth factor receptor (EGFR) conjugated to indocyanine for detection of human squamous cell carcinoma that were transplanted to nude mice were reported in 1992. Subsequently, the technology was used to detect precancerous mucosa in vivo in the hamster cheek pouch carcinogenesis model [44].

New therapeutic directions

The explosion of molecular targets that are implicated in squamous cell carcinoma (SCC) and that is afforded by the previously noted technologies is translated to targeted therapeutics for this disease. Undoubtedly, this trend will continue as specific means of targeting these molecules proceed from the bench to the bedside.

Epidermal growth factor receptor

EGFR is a tyrosine kinase receptor that is overexpressed in 80% to 100% of premalignant and malignant oral lesions [45,46]. When a ligand binds to the receptor, two molecules of the bound receptor bind and autophosphorylation occurs; this activates the tyrosine kinase activity and generates intracellular sequelae. Autophosphorylation has been described in the unbound receptor in response to tobacco smoke components [47]. The observation that tyrosine kinase inhibitors may halt the progression of aneuploid premalignant lesions further implicates EGFR in tumor progression [48].

The implication of EGFR in oral squamous cell carcinoma has led to the clinical use of various agents to block the function of this protein in the treatment of oral cancer. Two monoclonal antibodies C225/cetuximab (Erbitux, Imclone, New York, New York) and ZD1839/gefitinib (Iressa, Astra-Zeneca, London, UK) have been evaluated as therapeutic agents for oral carcinoma.

Gefitinib has been noted to halt proliferation and cause G1 phase cell cycle arrest [49] and to reduce regional nodal metastases [50] in oral squamous cell carcinoma (OSCC) xenografts in mice. Similarly, cetuximab was noted to promote G1 phase arrest in cultured OSCC cells [51]. Exposure to gefitinib also increased the radiosensitivity of OSCC cells in vitro and in vivo [52].

Vascular endothelial growth factor

The term angiogenesis refers to the creation of new microvasculature by a tumor to quench the metabolic demands of the tumor. Antiangiogenesis treatment modalities have been heralded as a great breakthrough in cancer therapeutics. Many methods of inhibiting angiogenesis have been proposed, including inhibition of matrix metalloproteinases, blockade of vascular endothelial growth factor (VEGF) and its receptor, and integrin blockade. Thalidomide was noted to have antiangiogenesis activity, and is being evaluated for use in this context.

In recent years, antiangiogenic therapies have been studied in clinical trials for tumors, such as lung cancer, colorectal cancer, and pancreatic cancer. With regard to head and neck tumors, VEGF has been the primary target. The expression of VEGF is increased significantly in invasive head and neck SCC compared with carcinoma in situ, dysplasia, and normal epithelium [53]. The treatment of head and neck SCC cell lines with antisense oligonucleotides that target VEGF mRNA decreased VEGF expression and endothelial migration [54,55] This treatment resulted in a significant decrease in VEGF protein expression and tumor growth in mice that had SCC xenografts [54].

Personalized therapy

Microarray cDNA library analysis allows measurement of expression of tens of thousands of genes by cancer cells; however, only a handful of these genes and their products has been studied as therapeutic targets. Further basic science and clinical experience will elucidate which of these genes will materialize as clinically significant. In the near future, one can envision a treatment program of 10 or even 100 monoclonal antibody-based agents as determined by microarray analysis of the individual tumor.

Summary

Future developments in the realms of nanotechnology and directed therapeutics will alter the diagnosis and treatment of oral cancer relative to contemporary treatment modalities. Continued experience and investigation will determine the clinical usefulness of the various technologies that have been described in this article.

References

[1] American Cancer Society. Cancer facts and figures, 2002. Atlanta (GA): American Cancer Society; 2002.
[2] Feynman R. There's plenty of room at the bottom. Science 1991;254:1300–1.
[3] National Nanotechnology Initiative.Available at: http://www.nano.gov/. Accessed August 15, 2005.
[4] The National Research Council Report. Small wonders, endless frontiers. Washington, DC: National Academy Press; 2000.
[5] Gao X, Cui Y, Levenson RM, et al. In vivo cancer targeting and imaging with semiconductor quantum dots. Nat Biotechnol 2004;22:969–76.
[6] Han M, Gao X, Su JZ, et al. Quantum-dot-tagged microbeads for multiplexed optical coding of biomolecules. Nat Biotechnol 2001;19:631–5.
[7] Chan WCW, Nie S. Quantum dot bioconjugates for ultrasensitive nonisotopic detection. Science 1998;281:2016–8.
[8] Akerman ME, Chan WCW, Laakkonen P, et al. Nanocrystal targeting in vivo. Proc Natl Acad Sci U S A 2002;99:12617–21.
[9] Dahan M. Diffusion dynamics of glycine receptors revealed by single quantum dot tracking. Science 2003;302:442–6.
[10] Bohren CF, Huffman DR. Absorption and scattering of light by small particles. New York: Wiley; 1983.

[11] Dirix Y, Bastiaansen C, Caseri W, et al. Oriented pearl-necklace arrays of metallic nanoparticles in polymers: a new route toward polarization-dependent color filters. Adv Mater 1999; 11:223–7.

[12] Csáki A, Kaplanek P, Möller R, et al. The optical detection of individual DNA-conjugated gold nanoparticle labels after metal enhancement. Nanotechnology 2003;14:1262–8.

[13] Sato T, Hasko DG, Ahmed H. Nanoscale colloidal particles: monolayer organization and patterning. J Vac Sci Technol B 1997;15:45–8.

[14] Nie S, Emory SR. Probing single molecules and single nanoparticles by surface-enhanced Raman scattering. Science 1997;275:1102–6.

[15] Brown KR, Walter DG, Natan MJ. Seeding of colloidal Au nanoparticle solutions. 2. Improved control of particle size and shape. Chem Mater 2000;12:306–13.

[16] Halas N. Optical properties of nanoshells. Opt Photonics News 2002;Aug:26–30.

[17] Aden AL, Kerker M. Scattering of electromagnetic waves from two concentric spheres. J Appl Phys 1951;22:1242–6.

[18] Zhou HS, Honma I, Komiyama H, et al. Controlled synthesis and quantum size effect in gold-coated nanoparticles. Phys Rev B 1994;50:12052–6.

[19] Averitt RD, Sarkar D, Halas NJ. Plasmon resonance shifts of Au-coated Au_2S nanoshells: insight into multicomponent nanoparticle growth. Phys Rev Lett 1997;78:4217–20.

[20] Oldenburg SJ, Averitt RD, Westcott SL, et al. Nanoengineering of optical resonances. Chem Phys Lett 1998;288:243–7.

[21] Stober W, Fink A, Bohn E. Controlled growth of monodisperse silica spheres in the micron size range. J Colloid Interface Sci 1968;26:62–9.

[22] Graf C, van Blaaderen A. Metallodielectric colloidal core-shell particles for photonic applications. Langmuir 2002;18:524–34.

[23] Duff DG, Baiker A, Edwards PP. A new hydrosol of gold clusters. 1. Formation and particle size variation. Langmuir 1993;9:2301–9.

[24] Duff DG, Baiker A, Edwards PP. A new hydrosol of gold clusters. 2. Comparison of some different measurement techniques. Langmuir 1993;9:2310–7.

[25] Sershen S, Westcott SL, Halas NJ, et al. Temperature-sensitive polymer-nanoshell composites for photothermally modulated drug delivery. J Biomed Mat Res 2000;51:293–8.

[26] Hirsch LR, Stafford RJ, Bankson JA, et al. Nanoshell-mediated near-infrared thermal therapy of tumors under magnetic resonance guidance. Proc Natl Acad Sci USA 2003;100:13549–54.

[27] Krauss W, editor. Contrast Agents I. Topics in current chemistry, vol. 221. New York: Springer; 2002.

[28] Moralesa MP, Bomati-Miguela O, Perez de Alejob R, et al. Contrast agents for MRI based on iron oxide nanoparticles prepared by laser pyrolysis. J Magn Magn Mater 2003;266:102–9.

[29] Kim DK, Mikhaylova M, Wang FH, et al. Starch-coated superparamagnetic nanoparticles as MR contrast agents. Chem Mater 2003;15:1543–51.

[30] Mornet S, Vasseur S, Grasset F, et al. Magnetic nanoparticle design for medical diagnosis and therapy. J Mater Chem 2004;14:2161–75.

[31] Lee S-J, Jeong J-R, Shin S-C, et al. Nanoparticles of magnetic ferric oxides encapsulated with poly(D, L latide-co-glycolide) and their applications to magnetic resonance imaging contrast agent. J Magn Magn Mater 2004;272–276:2432–3.

[32] Hergta R, Hiergeista R, Hilgerb I, et al. Magnemite nanoparticles with very high AC-losses for application in RF-magnetic hyperthermia. J Magn Magn Mater 2004;270:345–51.

[33] Imani F. Bioinformatics in otolaryngology. Otolaryngol Clin North Am 2005;38:321–32.

[34] Whipple ME, Mendez E, Farwell DG, et al. A genomic predictor of oral squamous cell carcinoma. Laryngoscope 2004;113:1346–54.

[35] Mendez E, Cheng C, Farwell DG, et al. Transcription expression profiles of oral squamous cell carcinomas. Cancer 2002;95:1482–94.

[36] Warner GC, Reis PP, Jurisica I, et al. Molecular classification of oral cancer by cDNA microarrays identifies overexpressed genes correlated with nodal metastasis. Int J Cancer 2004; 110:857–68.

[37] Schmalbach CE, Chepeha DB, Giordano TJ. Molecular profiling and identification of the genes associated with metastatic oral cavity/pharynx squamous cell carcinoma. Arch Otolaryngol Head Neck Surg 2004;130:295–302.

[38] Nagata M, Fujita H, Ida H, et al. Identification of potential biomarkers of lymph node metastasis in oral squamous cell carcinoma by cDNA microarray analysis. Int J Cancer 2003; 106:683–9.

[39] Belbin TJ, Singh B, Barber I, et al. Molecular classification of head and neck squamous cell carcinomas using cDNA microarrays. Cancer Res 2002;62:1184–90.

[40] Dhingra JK, Zhang X, McMillan K, et al. Diagnosis of head and neck precancerous lesions in an animal model using fluorescence spectroscopy. Laryngoscope 1998;108:471–5.

[41] Gillenwater A, Jacob R, Ganeshappa R, et al. Noninvasive diagnosis of oral neoplasia based on fluorescence spectroscopy and native tissue autofluorescence. Arch Otolaryngol Head Neck Surg 1998;124:1251–8.

[42] Chen CT, Chiang HK, Chow SN, et al. Autofluorescence in normal and malignant human oral tissues and in DMBA-induced hamster buccal pouch carcinogenesis. J Oral Pathol Med 1998;27:470–4.

[43] Folli S, Wagnieres G, Pelegrin A, et al. Immunophotodiagnosis of colon carcinomas in patients injected with fluoresceinated chimeric antibodies against carcinoembryonic antigen. Proc Natl Acad Sci U S A 1992;89:7973–7.

[44] Soukos NS, Hamblin MR, Keel S, et al. Epidermal growth factor receptor-targeted immunophotodiagnosis and photomimmunotherapy in oral precancer in vivo. Cancer Res 2001; 61:4490–6.

[45] Grandis JR, Tweardy DJ. Elevated levels of transforming growth factor alpha and epidermal growth factor receptor messenger RNA are early markers of carcinogenesis in head and neck cancer. Cancer Res 1993;53:3579–84.

[46] Shin DM, Ro JY, Hong WK, et al. Dysregulation of epidermal growth factor expression in premalignant lesions in head and neck tumorigenesis. Cancer Res 1994;54:3153–9.

[47] Dannenberg AJ, Lippman SM, Mann JR, et al. Cyclooxygenase-2 and epidermal growth factor receptor: pharmacologic targets for chemoprevention. J Clin Oncol 2005;23:254–66.

[48] Lippman SM, Sudbo J, Hong WK. Oral cancer prevention and the evolution of molecular-targeted drug development. J Clin Oncol 2005;23:346–56.

[49] Shintani S, Li C, Mihara M, et al. Gefitinib ('Iressa', ZD1839), an epidermal growth factor receptor tyrosine kinase inhibitor, up-regulates p27KIP1 and induces GI arrest in oral squamous cell carcinoma cell lines. Oral Oncol 2004;40:43–51.

[50] Shintani S, Li C, Mihara M, et al. Gefitinib ('Iressa'), an epidermal growth factor receptor tyrosine kinase inhibitor, mediates the inhibition of lymph node metastasis in oral cancer cells. Cancer Lett 2003;201:149–55.

[51] Kiyota A, Shintani S, Mihara M, et al. Anti-epidermal growth factor receptor monoclonal antibody 225 upregulates p27(KIP1) and p15(INK4B) and induces G1 arrest in oral squamous carcinoma cell lines. Oncology 2002;63:92–8.

[52] Harari PM, Huang SM. Head and neck cancer as a clinical model for molecular targeting of therapy: combining EGFR blockade with radiation. Int J Radiat Oncol Biol Phys 2001;49: 427–33.

[53] Sauter ER, Nesbit M, Watson JC. Vascular endothelial growth factor is a marker of tumor invasion and metastasis in squamous cell carcinomas of the head and neck. Clin Cancer Res 1999;5:775–82.

[54] Riedel F, Gotte K, Hormann K, et al. Antiangiogenic therapy of head and neck squamous cell carcinoma by vascular endothelial growth factor antisense therapy. Adv Otorhinolaryngol 2005;62:103–20.

[55] Nakashima T, Hudson JM, Clayman GL. Antisense inhibition of vascular endothelial growth factor in human head and neck squamous cell carcinoma. Head Neck 2000;22:483–8.

ELSEVIER
SAUNDERS

Otolaryngol Clin N Am
39 (2006) 397–402

OTOLARYNGOLOGIC
CLINICS
OF NORTH AMERICA

Index

Note: Page numbers of article titles are in **boldface** type.

0030-6665/06/$ - see front matter © 2006 Elsevier Inc. All rights reserved.
doi:10.1016/S0030-6665(06)00041-7   *oto.theclinics.com*

Changing Your Address?

Make sure your subscription changes too! When you notify us of your new address, you can help make our job easier by including an exact copy of your Clinics label number with your old address (see illustration below.) This number identifies you to our computer system and will speed the processing of your address change. Please be sure this label number accompanies your old address and your corrected address—you can send an old Clinics label with your number on it or just copy it exactly and send it to the address listed below.

We appreciate your help in our attempt to give you continuous coverage. Thank you.

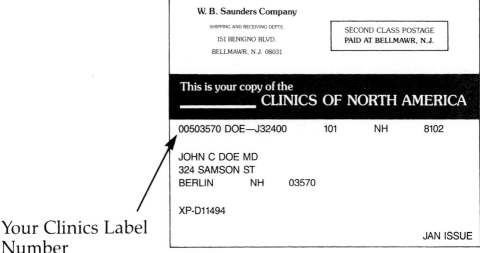

W. B. Saunders Company

SHIPPING AND RECEIVING DEPTS.
151 BENIGNO BLVD.
BELLMAWR, N.J. 08031

SECOND CLASS POSTAGE
PAID AT BELLMAWR, N.J.

This is your copy of the
_____ **CLINICS OF NORTH AMERICA**

00503570 DOE—J32400   101   NH   8102

JOHN C DOE MD
324 SAMSON ST
BERLIN   NH   03570

XP-D11494

JAN ISSUE

Your Clinics Label Number
Copy it exactly or send your label
along with your address to:
Elsevier Periodicals Customer Service
6277 Sea Harbor Drive
Orlando, FL 32887-4800
Call Toll Free 1-800-654-2452

Please allow four to six weeks for delivery of new subscriptions and for processing address changes.